THE TOXIC
DENTAL
OFFICE

HOW TO PROTECT
YOURSELF AND
YOUR FAMILY

THE TOXIC DENTAL OFFICE

HOW TO PROTECT YOURSELF AND YOUR FAMILY

Donald Robbins DMD

BRIGHTMARK

Exton, Pennsylvania

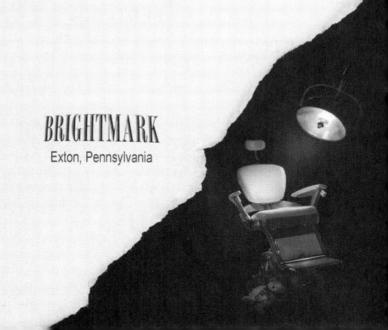

FIRST EDITION

Cover design and publication consultation by Robert Buckland
www.oceancooperative.com

Text design and layout by Jean Shepherd
jean.shepherd@videotron.ca

THE TOXIC DENTAL OFFICE
How to Protect Yourself and Your Family

Dr. Donald Robbins

ISBN 978-0-9824399-0-6

Printed in Canada

BRIGHTMARK

Acknowledgments

The author wishes to express thanks to those who have helped get this book to the public arena and who helped promote BioSafeDentistry® as the safe manner to practice dentistry in the 21st century. I especially wish to thank my wife, Kathleen Boyle, for her constant encouragement and constructive suggestions during the organization and writing and my editor, Robert Buckland, for his expressed passion to deliver this information to the public and for support organizing the manuscript for easy reading.

Professionally, I appreciate the training I received in dental school that allowed me to review all the scientific facts to make an informed, evidence-based decision on dental-health questions and treatment. The International Academy of Oral Medicine and Toxicology has been invaluable over the last seven years educating me beyond what I learned in dental school, and opening my eyes to a better, healthier way to practice dentistry. Appreciation is offered for the support given by Charlie Brown, national counsel of Consumers for Dental Choice, and Robert Reeves, attorney, for their encouragement to take career risks in the interest of helping individuals make informed decisions about their healthcare and for improving the status of medical and dental care.

I wish to thank my dental practice staff for enthusiastically supporting my BioSafeDentistry program and helping inform and educate my patients about their dental care and the choices they must make. Special thanks are extended to my office manager, Nina, who brought me to understand certain aspects of communication and how to interact with people in a better, more constructive way.

Lastly, let me thank all my friends who have seen very little of me over the last two years while this book was being researched and written.

Please let us all strive to improve our health care without regard to selfish financial gain or political power plays. To live to be 150 years old, we must look at the science and not censor new ideas.

Introduction

I've been a dentist for more than 30 years. During those decades I've spoken to thousands of patients who needed, feared, appreciated, loathed and questioned dental care. But it was only in the early '80s that I realized that the public is generally misinformed about what a dentist should be. Many patients—maybe most patients—see their dentist as a person who is always right. In fact, a good dentist acts first and foremost as a guide to your health-care choices and keeps an eye on your overall well-being. A good dentist's greater knowledge is there to help *you* choose.

That's why I wrote this book. I want to empower you to take control of your own health care, specifically your oral health, which will in turn affect your physical and emotional health. I'll tell you what you need to know: When you need to change dentists. When you need to ask questions. When you need to demand answers. And how to find a good dental practice in the first place.

As the years went on it became obvious to me, and many intuitive and progressive dentists, that our oral health reflects and affects the rest of our bodies. Diabetes has a profound effect on healing rates in the mouth. The same bacteria found in the inflamed and infected gum tissue associated with periodontal (gum) disease can cause cardiac myopathy and heart attacks. Stomach acids can eat away tooth structure and permanently damage teeth. Depression and neuroses can cause neglect of oral hygiene and subsequent decay.

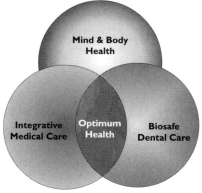

The circle diagram at the right, called a Venn diagram, illustrates the principles by which I practice. BioSafeDentistry™ is the term I use to describe integrative biologic dental care that uses biocompatible materials in a safe office environment where treatment is designed to maintain and restore physical and mental health. BioSafeDentistry integrates dental care with other aspects of health, both body and mind, to improve the patient's overall wellness.

Throughout this book I cite respected scientific journals and studies to support my statements. These are statements of fact that many dentists have never been exposed to. These statements may be viewed as inflammatory because the general public and the media (and many dentists) have been kept so long in the dark. My hope is that you, by reading The Toxic Dentist Office, *will learn the truth about real health dangers and how you can protect yourself and your families.*

Foreword

A MILL SLOWLY TURNING
I received this e-mail October 21, 2006.

> City: Mohnton
>
> State: PA
>
> HELP! I am 12 weeks pregnant and am 43 years old. This is
> our first child, coming unexpectedly. J and I recently read an
> article about mercury fillings causing autism in unborn
> children or even later on. I have about six and have upwards of
> 10 mercury fillings in my mouth. Is my baby truly at risk and
> is there anything I can do to protect it now. I appreciate any
> help you can give me, I am very worried!!
>
> Thank you.

On October 14, 2004, a bill was introduced in the Committee on
Licenses and Inspections, City Council of the City of Philadelphia,
requiring

> dentists to post and distribute certain information concerning
> the use of mercury in dental procedures, and requiring dentists
> to install systems that permit the recycling of mercury waste,
> all under certain terms and conditions.

The provisions of this bill allowed the public at large and the dental
patient in particular to know the facts about mercury. The bill required a booklet or placard to be placed in all general dental offices
in the City of Philadelphia. It would explain that patients must give
their informed consent to dental procedures involving mercury. Alternatively, patients may choose one of several alternative treatments
available. Failure to post such a notice would be tantamount to con-
cealing information from the public.

A further provision would require every dentist in Philadelphia to
install and use a mercury separator. Such devices, which remove
toxic mercury particles and sludge from the wastewater before it
goes into the municipal sewage system, are increasingly required by

municipalities elsewhere.

Political interests delayed the bill for three years.

On May 30, 2007, a meeting of the Council on Licenses and Inspections was scheduled at Philadelphia City Hall, City Council Chambers. I was called by the sponsors to testify on behalf of the stalled bill—the only dentist to do so.

A court official read a brief introduction of the proposed ordinance for the record. I looked around. There were representatives of consumer organizations, environmental groups and various city departments including the Philadelphia Health Department and, of course, three members of the Pennsylvania Dental Association. Each representative rose to speak on behalf of the bill. Then the Pennsylvania Dental Association dentists were called to give a statement.

"There's nothing wrong with mercury in the mouth," they protested. "It's been used for over 100 years with no problems and nobody gets sick from dental fillings." They wanted the committee to understand that there were no scientific studies to prove mercury dental fillings were dangerous. They argued that in some dental situations mercury amalgam fillings *must* be used to restore a tooth. If the patient's mouth cannot be kept dry, they warned, if there's too much saliva or water present, only mercury fillings will work. Then, perhaps concerned that their unsupported case might not carry the day, they added something astounding: "It would be a financial hardship for dentists to install and maintain mercury separators in their offices."

I sat back in my seat and made a groan that may have been audible. Around me, I saw other expert witnesses rolling their eyes. The dental establishment had been talking this line for generations, in effect preventing progressive dental care from improving the health of the public. I could hardly believe that these people were still prepared, at this point in history, and with public awareness of mercury rising, to trot out the same shopworn arguments. None of their claims could be supported by reputable, unbiased scientific studies. And as to placing a filling in a patient's mouth if the tooth was wet—apparently organized dentistry's attempt to put a technical issue over on the public and the first time I'd seen this card played in testimony—no dental school on the continent would condone such sloppy technique. Any student in any dental school who tried to place a filling in a tooth improperly prepared would get an automatic failing grade. Dentistry is surgery, surgery that cannot heal itself if performed improperly. There's no room for incompetent technique.

When I was called, I took a seat at the microphone and demonstrated that the Pennsylvania Dental Association was selling the committee a bill of goods. There was not one iota of truth in most of the statements the association's representatives were putting forward. I cited huge epidemiological studies and reviews by the United States Department of Health and Human Services, the US Environmental Protection Agency and the World Health Organization performed from 1991 through the present. These studies support the toxicity of mercury in dental fillings and, alas, in dentists themselves. I cited the US Food and Drug Administration hearings from September 2006, in which the FDA convened expert panels to review the question of the neurotoxicity of mercury amalgam dental fillings. The FDA found they could not certify dental mercury amalgam fillings as safe. I reminded the committee that the dentist was responsible not just to the patient but to the environment. I explained to the committee that I had just paid $17,000 for a dental chair and unit. For the Pennsylvania Dental Association to claim that a $500 to $1500 one-time cost for a mercury separator constituted a *hardship* for dentists was absurd, bordering on obscene. "The dentist," I reminded them, "is responsible not just to the patient but has a civic responsibility to the environment as well."

I informed the committee members that the tendency of old and stubborn dentists is to intentionally fail to mention the mercury issue to their patients. This bill required dentists to discuss with patients the alternative non-mercury treatments available. Now I urged the committee to add a provision to the bill that would require the informed and signed consent of pregnant women, nursing mothers and the guardians of children before they could be subjected to mercury procedures.

I impressed upon the committee that the general public is concerned about the mercury in dental fillings and I read aloud the e-mail at the top of this chapter. I receive such e-mails almost daily, especially from patients with special medical issues. The public simply doesn't know where to turn for objective answers to the question of mercury in dental fillings. As things stand, old-fashioned dentists are making health-related choices for their patients without the patients' knowledge or consent. This bill, I pleaded, was necessary to assure that patents are educated about their health decisions.

The Committee on Licenses and Inspections voted and passed the bill onto the full city council hearing. On December 13, 2007, by a vote of 17 to 0, the bill was adopted by the City Council. This bill constitutes a turning point in the fight for informed consent for patients. The Pennsylvania Dental Association pleaded so strongly that it would cost dentists too much money to install amalgam separators that the City Council allowed that section of the "Mercury in Dentistry" bill to be removed. The people of the City of Philadelphia are still paying for the removal of mercury from their public water supply—mercury that comes from private dental offices.

This meeting of one committee in the administration of one municipality may seem insignificant in itself. But it joins many other such meetings as witness to a broad wave of change that is gathering momentum and is about to sweep through the field of dentistry, not just here in North America but around the world. Mercury, I'm afraid, is only a part of the story. In the course of this book, I'm going to bring you inside the profession so you'll be better able to appreciate not just what's coming, but how it happened that untold thousands of well-meaning professionals have perpetrated a public health menace, endangered the patients they wanted to help, and been controlled as patsies by political forces of breathtaking cynicism.

You might have hesitated to pick this book from the shelves. You might well be expecting to doubt what you're about to read. You've got a feeling maybe that you've heard all this sometime, somewhere before. If you're over, say, 30, and certainly if you're over 50, you'll remember various alarms about mercury, and especially about the fluoridation of water. You might still retain some faint memory of how those who opposed these pillars of mainstream dentistry were finally exposed as a radical fringe element—kooks and cranks. It was all quite a while ago, right?

But as it turns out, the truth has been the pea in a long-running shell game and like all shell games, the pea shufflers—in this case, bureaucrats and politicians—won in the short run. What you may *not* have heard is that, since then, the relentless advance of peer-reviewed science has lifted the shells and discovered the pea was missing altogether. This time around, the kooks and cranks turned out to be right.

But don't take my word for it. This book is about the work of many people. I make a contribution here and there, but more than anything else, I'm here to lay out the results of the hard—and some-times courageous—work of many others. It was work worth doing and it's work worth reading about. The truth must often bide its time. Like justice, its wheel turns slowly but it grinds exceeding small.

A Note to My Colleagues

I love my profession. It's my route to personal satisfaction and, like all medicine, it offers the reward of helping others. I'm sure you feel the same.

It's not our fault if we didn't have all the information. Our colleagues in the medical profession bled their patients white until 100 years ago. They'd been taught that bleeding was effective and it was the rare physician for whom observation alone could change their thinking and their actions in spite of received wisdom. Our work is critical and performed in the present. We must proceed with the tools we have and we now have plenty.

Questions of fault arise when we *do* have the information but choose to disregard it. In this respect, each healer is to some degree on his own. Change comes slowly and there is often a significant lag between the emergence of knowledge and its enforcement by statute or consensus. During that grey interval, innovations may be exposed as errors or confirmed as the real thing. We each struggle to decide.

In recent centuries, medicine has become more and more an applied branch of science, and we practitioners have become more and more obliged to seek out the truth. Knowledge pours in from every side, but we can't escape by shutting our eyes and ears and repeating over and over what we were taught when we were young.

If your dental practice today employs some of the outdated materials and techniques exposed in this book, I want you to know that I once shared your view. It was only professional curiosity, and the desire to improve my patients' health, that led me to lift the shells and look underneath for the pea of truth. But once I'd seen that truth, there was no going back. My reversal on various issues might have been embarrassing—there was always the possibility in a litigious society that I might attract a private suit for not changing sooner—but there could be no going back. I owed it to myself, of course, and I owed it to the patients who had placed their trust in me. Doctor, first do no harm.

Donald Robbins
Exton, Pennsylvania, January, 2009

Contents

1
MERCURY

"What good is informed consent if patients are not told what they need to know about their treatment?"

~ Councilwoman Blondell Reynolds Brown
City Hall
Philadelphia, Pa.

Appearances often obscure the true nature of things and some skepticism is healthy—a survival strategy. I'm going to make some harsh critiques of the dental profession in this book, but the fact remains that most dentists have a true desire to improve and preserve their patients' dental health, indeed their overall health. But the simple yet carefully obscured truth is that modern dental education has been manipulated to protect the interests of certain groups who have a vested interest in the status quo.

❧

Janice had just driven 175 miles from northern New Jersey to consult with me. She had tried the previous month to talk again to a dentist in her neighborhood about the mercury in her silver fillings.

"We don't use any mercury in the new fillings we put in teeth," he'd assured her. "We only use white, bonded fillings. We recommend removing the old black mercury fillings patients still have in their mouths, and bonding these new resin materials in the tooth instead."

But how did they remove the mercury fillings, she wanted to know.

The dentist had smiled. "No problem. We give you Novacaine and just drill out the old amalgam. You won't feel a thing."

"But what protection do you take so I don't get exposed to the mercury that comes off when you drill them out?"

The dentist was still thinking about an answer as Janice left the office.

She'd done her homework. She wasn't going to get sick again. Two years before her appointment in New Jersey, she began to be concerned about the mercury exposure from the many silver-mercury fillings in her teeth. She'd gone initially to a "holistic" dentist for the removal and replacement of her amalgam mercury fillings. The dentist she chose, if he had been truly knowledgeable in biologic dentistry, would have known how to safely remove and replace amalgam mercury fillings. He didn't. He removed two of her mercury fillings and placed two bonded composite resin fillings, but took no precautions to protect her—and himself and his staff—from the mercury vapor release. Within the first week Janice became ill. After seeing several physicians, her internist diagnosed "leaky gut syndrome"—a condition that increases the spaces between the intestinal cells, allowing them to pass bacteria, toxins and food from the gut into the bloodstream with little restrictions or protection. Since Janice had shown no symptoms of stomach or intestinal problems in the past, it was apparent she had reacted to the mercury exposure. She went on to suffer from chronic fatigue, muscle pains and weakness, and symptoms similar to irritable bowel syndrome (IBS)—abdominal pain, distension, diarrhea and bleeding. It took nearly two years of supportive treatment for her body to recover from the condition.

Now she knew what to look for in a dentist. She had come to my office after investigating many practices with websites on the internet. She knew I took maximum precautions to avoid mercury exposure. We eventually removed her remaining fillings safely and she experienced no further health consequences.

A Short History of Dentistry

When dentistry began to organize in the nineteenth century, dental snake oil and quackery were widespread. Unethical merchants sold whatever they could, and promised whatever the customer wanted to hear. Their products rarely produced the desired effect but—let the buyer beware!—the customer was out of luck and money. The practicing dentists of the time strove to elevate dental care to a respectable profession by improving dental care and investigating treatments to determine which were legitimate and which false.

In the United States, two men—Dr. Chapin A. Harris, a practicing physician who turned to dentistry in 1828, and Dr. Horace Henry Hayden, the first dentist to lecture on dentistry to medical students at the University of Maryland until 1825—led this movement. In 1840 they founded the first dental school in the world, the Baltimore College of Dental Surgery and the nation's first national dental organization, The American Society of Dental Surgeons, founded upon scientific and medical principles. At the time there were only about 300 trained and scientific dentists practicing in the country. The Society deemed the rest to be quacks and charlatans.

I'm afraid the following will shock you. Society members were *required* to sign a mandatory pledge not to use mercury fillings for fear of causing mercury poisoning in patients. Members of the society were suspended if they were found to be using mercury fillings. In his opening address to the first class of the Baltimore College of Dental Surgery in 1840, Dr. Harris had this to say about mercury dental fillings:

> It is one of the most objectionable articles for filling teeth that can be employed, and yet from the wonderful virtues ascribed to this pernicious compound by those who used it, thousands were induced to try its efficacy.

"Those who used it" were the flim-flam men of their time. They promised amazing results that were unfounded and dangerous. In some instances, the offending dentist was prosecuted for injury to the patient. According to E. S. Talbot, writing in the *Ohio State Journal of Dental Science* in 1882, the placement of mercury fillings in the teeth were shown in some cases to cause general nerve toxicity and the death of the unfortunate patient.

So how *could* this poisonous material survive for over 150 years as an accepted dental restorative material? How could all these altruistic dentists, aware of the science and physiology of mercury poisoning, and aware of how serious the damaging effects of mercury were for patients, allow the continued use of this material in their dental practices?

They Followed the Money

There were few alternatives to mercury amalgam for filling teeth until relatively recently. The only dependable alternative for many decades were gold restorations, expensive and short-lived. Amalgam was cheap, easy and fast to place in the tooth and it lasted a reasonable length of time in service. Patients have short memories and a few years later, when the tooth broke or became infected, they would not make the connection to the use of a filling material placed years previously. Dentists began using amalgam because that was how they were able to make money and stay in business. Pressure for dentists to place these easy and profitable fillings was so intense that in 1850, the Society *reversed its position and rescinded the no-amalgam pledge.* This was not based on any science or medical review of patients who became sick. It was based purely on political pressure: use anything to fill teeth—*but fill the teeth.* In 1859 the controversy resulted in the disbanding of the American Society of Dental Surgeons.

That very year, from the ashes of this ethical society, arose the American Dental Association (ADA). To no one's surprise, the new ADA did not forbid the use of amalgam in the mouth; indeed they were its principle advocate. From 1859 until 1984, the ADA has stubbornly maintained that the mercury in dental amalgam, about half the total filling material, is somehow different from mercury elsewhere. No scientific evidence supports this position either, yet the Association still trumpets the safety of the material on the grounds that the mercury is solidly bound in the dental filling material and not released into the body. This was known to be untrue over 150 years ago. It remains a deception today.

A Short History of the Tannery Industry

Almost everyone has read Lewis Carroll's *Alice in Wonderland* or at least seen a movie or cartoon based on its story. One of the most memorable scenes is the Mad Hatter's tea party.

The term "mad as a hatter" was current in the eighteenth century—well before Carroll's time. During this whole period, mercury was used in the manufacture of felt for hats, a process that entailed heating and stirring the liquid metal in large open vats. The workers could not avoid inhaling the vapors, which in due course caused neurological disorders such as confused speech, walking problems and distorted vision and eye movements.

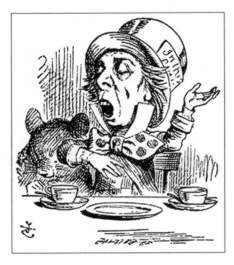

Figure 1-1: "The Hatter" after Tenniel (1865)

This would progress to abnormal behavioral changes such as violent outbursts and memory lapses. In those days any changes in public behaviors that deviated from the norm were termed "mad."

Today, these neurological symptoms, caused by the absorption of mercury through the skin or through inhalation, are termed Wernicke's encephalopathy. If allowed to continue, this condition can progress to Korsakoff's psychosis, a recent designation usually associated with chronic alcoholism and subsequent thiamine (B_1) deficiency. If untreated, the next stage can be brain damage in the form of permanent dementia such as Alzheimer's disease. I refer you to the Appendix A, page 266, for a list of symptoms of acute mercury poisoning.

SOURCES OF MERCURY EXPOSURE

Dental fillings are not the only source of mercury to which the average person is exposed. After all, mercury is found in the earth's crust in nearly every location. However, except for an environmental disaster, living next to a coal-burning power plant or receiving several injections of vaccines containing the mercury preservative thimerosal, dental amalgam fillings remain the biggest threat of mercury toxicity to humans. They continuously corrode in the mouth and off-gas mercury that is inhaled or absorbed into the body.

❧

Phillip ended up in my dental chair after consulting with five other dentists. He was a 29-year-old, post-graduate business student and was reading a textbook while waiting for me. He had a peculiar problem and I wasn't confident I could help him after five other dentists had failed.

"Whenever I brush my teeth I get a sick-to-my-stomach nauseous feeling for an hour or so," he explained. "I've tried changing toothpastes and toothbrushes but there was no difference. I'm sorry for the way my teeth look but it's hard to keep them clean without brushing more."

He looked dejected and a little embarrassed about his teeth. He probably felt the same way I did: there was little hope I could help after the other dentists could not.

I examined his mouth.

"You have quite a few mercury fillings in your teeth," I observed. "How long have they been there?"

"Most are five years or more."

"And how long has the nausea been affecting you?"

"It started about three to four years ago. Doc, the nausea is so bad I feel sick even when I get my teeth polished in a dentist's office."

I proceeded to test his oral mercury vapor levels with the atomic spectrometer I have in my office. Using atomic absorption technology, this device can measure mercury vapor to within 1 microgram per cubic meter. Phillip's test results were what I expected.

"The reading from your mouth at a resting level showed 1.2 micrograms per cubic meter of mercury vapor. You have 12 mercury filling surfaces in your mouth, in seven teeth. Understand that each tooth can have one to five surfaces restored with filling material. After you chewed the gum for three minutes, the reading was 10.6 micrograms per cubic meter."

The 1.2 level represented the level of mercury vapor that Phillip was exposed to 24 hours per day, seven days per week. This is relatively low. According to the US Environmental Protection Agency (US EPA), the maximum allowable inhalation level for which there is no evidence of noticeable health risk is 9 micrograms per cubic meter, an average for the general population. But the World Health Organization (WHO) in 1991 listed the only safe mercury exposure level as zero. Individuals exhibit more or less sensitivity to the metal. It is not possible to predict these individual reactions, so everyone must be protected.

According to the Michigan Health Department a *residence* can have no more than 1 microgram per cubic meter to protect pregnant women and children under six years of age.

Phillip and I looked together at the vapor-test results, especially the 10.6 reading.

"When you activate the surface of your mercury amalgam fillings by chewing, drinking hot beverages or carbonated sodas, or anything acidic like lemonade, the mercury vapor that's released increases dramatically. In your case it increased to 10.6. It then takes approximately an hour to an hour and a half to come back to the resting level.

"During that whole time you're being exposed to mercury vapor that you inhale or swallow. This mercury gets absorbed directly into your body and can make you feel sick and can have serious health effects on many of your body systems."

Phillip was closely following everything I was telling him.

"But what about the tooth brushing?" he asked.

"Good question. In my opinion, you're probably not a good excreter of mercury from your body. Some people genetically can excrete toxic heavy metals from their bodies faster. Your body probably has a much slower capability. The mercury lingers in your tissues and more become imbedded in tissues and cells. This makes it much harder to get it out of your body. It's probable that you are more sensitive to the effects of mercury than the average person.

"Now on top of that problem, when you brush your teeth you're *adding* even more mercury into your system by further activating the filling surfaces with your brushing and toothpaste. This additional mercury is immediately making you feel sick and nauseous.

"I can't guarantee that replacing the mercury fillings will stop the nausea, but it probably will. I *can guarantee* that getting those mercury-amalgam fillings out of your teeth will stop further off-gassing of mercury into your body. Long term health benefits are much improved without that additional toxic metal in your tissues."

There was no hesitation. Phillip agreed to have the seven mercury fillings removed safely and replaced with white bonded restorations. We took extra precautions to protect him from the extremely high mercury vapor that gets released when a filling is drilled out of a tooth. We didn't want to make his toxic absorption worse. Three months later he returned to my office for a routine scaling and polishing. He was smiling when I entered the hygienist's room.

"Doc, I really have to thank you! Since you got those fillings out I've been feeling great! I haven't had any sick feeling when I brush and I feel like I have a lot more energy. Thanks again!"

✑

We took another oral mercury vapor level reading that day. With no mercury dental fillings in his teeth, the results before and after chewing were now 0.0 and 1.0 micrograms per cubic meter.

When we review the effects of mercury in a later section, you'll see there are many different ways it disrupts the body's systems. Not everyone gets symptoms such as Phillip experienced, but most have their health affected in some harmful way, either in the short term or long term, or both. Except for an actual injection of mercury directly into the body with a needle (as with vaccines), the fastest way to absorb mercury is by inhaling it into the lungs where it immediately transfers to the blood stream. It only takes minutes before it is transformed into a fat soluble organic form and gets absorbed into the body, usually into the body fats and liver initially.

This is one reason why it is *extremely important* to have mercury amalgam fillings removed safely, with all precautions taken. Without these precautions, the considerable mercury vapor absorbed into the body during removal can have serious health consequences. The amount of mercury in the plasma, urine and blood have been measured immediately after simple removal without precautions and months after removal. Most show major increases in body levels of the toxic metal, which must then be removed by a physician trained in chelation and removal procedures. Even though some of these studies showed that several months (60-100 days) after the dental fillings were removed, the mercury levels in the body had decreased, these studies failed to take into account the mercury that had infiltrated body cells and systems during that time and so did not show up in a simple blood or urine test. This imbedded cellular mercury can be responsible for the symptoms of chronic mercury toxicity.

Some years ago, a bill to regulate the labelling of hazardous substances—including dental amalgam—remained tied up in the California state legislature. In 1986, the substance of this bill was placed on a ballot as Proposition 65 and subsequently passed. It was not proposed by the dental association. It was not proposed by the state legislature. The people of California voted to approve this informed consent for patients because they understood that mercury is toxic in any form. It was not until 2003, however, that a California Superior

Court judge finalized the language for a warning about the dangers of mercury in dental fillings that, for the first time anywhere, dentists would be required to post in their offices.

NOTICE TO PATIENTS

PROPOSITION 65 Warning: Dental Amalgams, used in many dental fillings, cause exposure to mercury, a chemical known to the state of California to cause birth defects or other reproductive harm.[1]

None of this is meant to minimize the effect that mercury from other sources can have on our lives and the environment. As everyone knows, it's politically acceptable to attack most other sources of mercury contamination on the basis of its toxic effects. But public assaults on mercury dental fillings as a source of toxicity exposure have been conspicuously few. We will soon examine why.

Let's review these other sources of mercury exposure.

Fertilizers

Mercurial compounds were used for decades in the manufacture of fertilizers, fungicides, mildewcides and pesticides, and included use in food crops. In 1969 the uses of mercury-containing pesticides were prohibited. All pesticide registrations were cancelled in 1995. The last four uses allowed were turf fungicide, mildewcide for fresh-cut wood, latex paint fungicide/preservative and outdoor fabric treatment; all were eventually cancelled. However, according to John Gilkeson, of the Minnesota Pollution Control Agency, some mercury-containing chemicals may still be present as old inventory, although they are not to be used today. He further reports that some mercury-containing pesticides are still being manufactured and used in other developed countries. For example, Canada still allows the

---

[1] Toxicological profile for mercury available at:
<http://www.atsdr1.atsdr.cdc.gov:8080/97list.html>,
<http://www.atsdr.cdc.gov/toxprofiles/tp46.pdf>

use of mercuric pesticides for turf mold. It is possible that mercury-containing pesticides are manufactured in the US for export.

Insecticides

Years ago I needed an exterminator because of an ant problem. He came into my office and began spraying around the baseboards of each room and then went outside to spray. I did not understand about toxicity from chemical sources in those days but I did ask him what he was spraying. He said it was some complicated chemical that "has mercury in it which kills the bugs but has a low enough concentration so it doesn't bother people." It was even odorless.

Today I know that these "harmless" toxic chemicals are not harmless at all. Even though they don't kill us like they kill the insects, they do accumulate in our bodies and can make us very sick. There are now better compounds to stop insects in our houses but you always have every right to know, and should know, *exactly* what they are spraying and what the effects are on people. The companies have a legal obligation to disclose any possible effects the sprayed chemicals might have on a susceptible person or pet animal.

We're all familiar with the use of canaries many years ago in coal mines to alert the miners if methane gas was creeping into the tunnels. The canaries would stop singing, even die, and this alerted the miners to get the heck out of the mine or (more recently) put on oxygen masks. You may remember a few years ago hearing stories about household birds falling mysteriously sick and dying as a result of the "harmless" Teflon™ coating on cookware. The suspected toxin was perfluorooctanoic acid (PFOA), used in the manufacture process of Teflon and emitted when the Teflon is heated. PFOA is a proven carcinogen, and when it builds up in the body it can cause cancer, liver damage and birth defects in animals. It has been found to be present in the blood of 95% of Americans including pregnant women. The Teflon-toxicity connection was eventually made. I hope the birds' owners got the message they themselves could become seriously toxic. If you are inclined to dismiss this as an urban myth, you should know that the use of Teflon in cookware, microwave popcorn bags and waterproof clothing will be stopped by 2015. This "ban" on Teflon is actually an agreement from eight chemical companies to voluntarily phase out its manufacture by 2015. DuPont was fined $16 million in December 2005 for hiding evidence of PFOA's toxicity, which the company was shown to know about. A related chemical, PFOS, was used by 3M Corporation to make Scotchguard™ products. In May 2000, in an agreement with the US Environmental Protection Avency (EPA), 3M agreed to halt its production as well.

> Dental amalgams…may represent the largest single non-occupational contributing source to total body burden of…mercury in people with…amalgam fillings.
> —*1999, The US Department of Health and Human Service, Atlanta, GA*

Fish

By now, everyone knows about the mercury contamination of fish. Little fish absorb a little mercury, usually from sludge at the bottom of the water. Bigger fish eat the little fishes and accumulate more mercury and so on. The large billfish such as swordfish and marlin at the top of the food chain eat all the other fish and have the most mercury in their tissues. What actually are those mercury levels?

Numerous studies of mercury levels in fish have been done by independent investigators and governmental and non-governmental agencies including the WHO (see Graph 1-1), the US Department of Health and Human Services (US HHS), the US Agency for Toxic Substances and Disease Registry (ATSDR) and others. If you want to know *exactly* how much mercury is in a particular fish, the United States Food and Drug Administration (US FDA) has a website listing all known species and the average mercury content of each.

There is a general consensus on the range of mercury absorbed daily by the general population. The estimated absorption of mercury from foods other than fish, air and water together is *0.3 micrograms per day*. The estimated absorption of mercury from all forms of fish and seafood is 2.34 micrograms per day.

According to all the studies outlined by WHO in 1991 and the US Department of Health and Human Services in 1999, the estimated daily absorption of mercury from an average number of *dental mercury fillings is 3 to 17 micrograms per day*.

Perhaps you'd like to read that last sentence again. *The mercury absorption from dental fillings may account for 87% of all daily absorbed mercury*. The alerts and news reports of pregnant women and children avoiding eating fish has merit but the media and government have failed to underline the major cause of mercury toxicity: *dental amalgam fillings*.

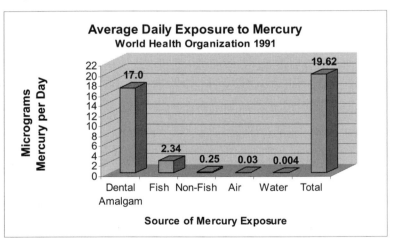

Graph 1-1: Absorption of mercury from dental fillings far exceeds mercury from any other daily source[2]

---

[2] *Environmental Health Criteria 118, Inorganic mercury.* 1991, US HHS, ATSDR, *Toxicological Profile For Mercury. 1999,* http://www.atsdr1.atsdr.cdc.gov:8080/97list.html, Zander, *Exposure to mercury in the population. II. Mercury release from amalgam fillings].* 1990

Coal Plants

A 2003 report by The Northeast States Coordinated Air Use Management (NESCAUM), a non-profit association of eight state departments of environmental protection, reports that US coal-fired power plants *"...are the largest unregulated sources of mercury emissions and are responsible for approximately 40 percent of the country's industrial emissions."* They estimate that ⅓ of all mercury deposition in the environment comes from power plants.

Technologies are available now to reduce mercury emissions by over 90% for power plants with costs comparable to current federal regulations for reducing ozone emissions. Technologies being developed promise to virtually eliminate toxic emissions from coal-burning plants. Getting states and federal agencies (and politicians, many of whose reelection campaigns rely on power companies' contributions) to require this commitment is the only real stumbling block.

Cremation

Each year more people are choosing cremation as the ultimate option. In 2003 there were nearly 700,000 cremations or 28.6 percent of deaths. The Cremation Association of North America estimates that by 2025 there will be 1.4 million cremations annually in North America—43 percent of the number of total deaths.

But—get ready for this—cremations add a significant mercury burden to the air, estimated by the New England Zero Mercury Campaign in 2005 to be 2.5 tons annually in the US alone. That mercury comes from the vaporization of dental mercury fillings in people's mouths during the procedure. By comparison, all this country's coal-burning power plants emitted only 48 tons that same year. But emissions from coal-burning plants are expected to decrease over the next 10 years or so as more stringent US EPA regulations come into effect. Emissions from cremations, meanwhile, are expected to rise and responsible agencies would be well advised to mandate further scientific studies that can evaluate this threat.

Global Environmental Recycling

These first five sources of mercury exposure are tightly interrelated environmentally. Figure 1-2 shows how mercury travels and moves from one source to another. Even the mercury we dispose of eventually finds its way back into the human sphere, either through the air, following the incineration of waste or, following the burial of waste, through underground water courses to rivers, lakes and oceans, from which it evaporates and finally falls again as contaminated rain. All three environmental components—air, water and earth—must be carefully regulated to avoid mercury contamination.

Recycling implies the collection of reusable environmental resources and making them available for use again after proper processing. But mercury is not a resource to be recycled because *there is no safe use for it.* Once it has been collected, we need more than anything to secure methods of storage so it cannot recontaminate our environment.

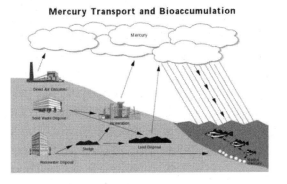

Figure 1-2: Mercury exposure from one source to another

Thermometers, Thermostats and Other Devices

In the past, mercury was used for many types of switches because, as a liquid, it seeks its own level under the influence of gravity and as a metal it can conduct electricity. Old heating and air conditioning thermostats used mercury to switch the systems on and off according to ambient room temperature. One study reveals that in 2001, in the US alone, over 28,000 pounds of mercury (13,000 kilograms) were sold in thermostats. Each thermostat contained 2,200 to 3,000 milligrams of elemental liquid mercury. This is an extremely dangerous source of mercury vapor in the home should these ampules fracture and the mercury be released to the air. Yet the EPA and other governmental agencies have only made it a *recommendation* through federal guidelines, that mercury thermostats be returned and recycled properly. The same is true of mercury thermometers. The silver colored liquid in glass thermometers is liquid mercury (any color other

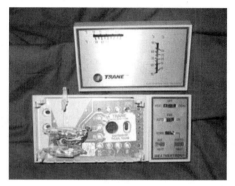

Figure 1-3: Old type of mercury thermostat. Note two glass vials of liquid mercury.

than silver is usually not liquid mercury). There are no federal requirements to phase out mercury thermometers, only a guideline and recommendation to safely turn them in to recycling centers and to use non-mercury thermometers instead. The typical thermometer contains between 0.5 and 3 grams of elemental liquid mercury— again, a potentially dangerous amount if released into the air. Both the American Academy of Pediatrics and the US EPA have been recommending and encouraging the discontinuance of mercury thermometers.

If everyone knows mercury is extremely harmful to people, why haven't thermometers, thermostats, and other products containing mercury been eliminated? Why hasn't mandatory recycling and return of these products been implemented? We can quite reasonably ask: Are some government agencies that were created to actively protect the public from toxic exposures failing to do so?

Dental Offices

Dentists who still place mercury amalgam fillings—and those who do not take safety precautions while removing old mercury fillings—expose everyone to mercury and potential toxicity. Drilling out an old mercury filling causes the inorganic mercury to aerosol and vaporize, raising the concentrations in the mouth and surrounding area from tens to hundreds of times its resting rate. This of course allows the patient to inhale and swallow large amounts of mercury. It also exposes the dentist and staff at chairside and those working anywhere in the office to a constant level. If no precautions are taken, the chronic release of mercury vapor and particulates contaminates room surfaces, actually getting into the surfaces of things like wallpaper, carpets and drapes, further increasing the concentration of mercury.

When patients walk into a dental office, they have no way of calculating the room level of mercury vapor they are inhaling. It's of utmost importance that you as a patient do your homework and choose a dental practice that knows about this issue and has taken steps to keep the office uncontaminated. I'm going to help you do that later in this book.

Tanneries

Mercury has not been used for tanning hides for many years. Chromium sulfate and tree bark tannins are now used in the semi-automatic tanning process. However there are many ground sites where tanneries once stood and the grounds (and any structures still standing) are still toxic with chemicals. These sites can remain contaminated and capable of seriously sickening anyone for many, many years, even centuries. Use of this ground for normal activities and construction necessitates a clean-up of the contaminated soil.

Vaccines with Thimerosal

For many years the organomercurial chemical thimerosal was used as a preservative in multi-dose vials of vaccines. The United States Code of Federal Regulations (CFR) in 1968 required preservatives be incorporated into the vaccines. Thimerosal is approximately 50% mercury and after injection is degraded to ethylmercury. A vaccine containing 0.01% thimerosal as a preservative contains approximately 25 micrograms of mercury per 0.5 ml dose.

Various agencies developed guidelines for what they considered a "safe" exposure to methylmercury. These exposure limits range from 0.1 micrograms/kg body wt/day (US EPA) to 0.47 micrograms/kg body wt/day (WHO). Concerns arose as the number of vaccines recommended for a child increased over the years, and with it an increased exposure to the mercury in thimerosal. After the US Congress asked the US National Academy of Sciences (NAS) to establish an official methylmercury minimal "safety" dose (RfD), the NAS reported that RfD was equal to the US EPA dose of 0.1 microgram/kg body wt/day.

In hearings and panel reviews in 1999 and 2000, the US FDA and the American Academy of Pediatrics issued two joint statements urging vaccine manufacturers to reduce or eliminate thimerosal in vaccines as soon as possible. This gives us little basis for comfort

1. There is no "safe" exposure level to mercury. The World Health Organization has declared the only safe level of mercury exposure is zero.

2. Twenty-five micrograms of mercury injected in a 0.5 ml dose is a lot of mercury injected right into your tissues with no regard for how it effects the neurological system or how well it is excreted by the specific patient, if at all.

3. By not making the elimination of mercury as thimerosal in vaccines mandatory, the US FDA allowed the vaccines still on the shelves to be used up first. This allowed the unnecessary exposure

of mercury as an injected toxin into children's bodies solely for the purpose of using up old vaccine. A mandatory ban on all the vaccines on the shelves containing mercury preservatives would have meant all these old vials would have been recalled, an expensive proposition for the manufacturers. Children were in effect poisoned to satisfy adult greed.

The Good News. As of 2007, no pediatric vaccines have thimerosal as a preservative in them except for some of the influenza (flu) vaccines.

The Bad News. I believe that thimerosal and mercury contributed to the development of autism and other neurological and learning disorders in thousands of children. We will be dealing with the aftermath of this toxic exposure for decades to come.

The Other Bad News. Many adult vaccines still contain mercury as a preservative. There does not appear to be any big rush by the US FDA to require universal removal of thimerosal from these vaccines, and a mandatory recall of old vials. Those vaccines with live attenuated cultures (measles, mumps and rubella vaccine (MMR), varicella) need not be recalled because they cannot contain thimerosal, which would kill the medically active organisms.

⟨ℚ

At the time of this story, my wife, Kathleen, was in her 30s, single, and did a lot of international traveling for her job. She lived in an apartment when in town, which was about 60% of the time. She suffered from severe food allergies and had passed out several times when exposed to shellfish.

Kathleen traveled frequently to Great Britain, regularly staying at a hotel two hours outside London. Her trips were usually five to 12 days and occurred throughout the year. One particular trip was longer and took place during the summer. Many living facilities in Britain do not have air conditioning due to the generally cool climate, and they rely on open windows and fresh-air ventilation. Such was the case at Kathy's hotel. However, during the first week she developed a rash on her legs which gradually got worse. She had difficulty breathing during exertion and felt generally weak and sick. She got so bad that the local doctors were afraid of letting her fly home for fear of a health emergency occurring on the plane during the long flight. Once at home she consulted with several physicians, and took a battery of tests. Her blood tests revealed serious liver dysfunction, with her liver enzymes almost eight times the level they should be.

She made an appointment with a nationally prominent liver specialist in Philadelphia. The specialist reviewed her test results and informed her that she had idiopathic hepatitis, that is, a severe inflammation of the liver with no known cause. He told her the enzyme levels were so bad she had only six months to two years, at best, to live.

"If you do exactly what I tell you to do and take medication as I prescribe, you may live longer." That was his advice. "I recommend a liver biopsy, but it is a dangerous procedure and there is a slight risk of dying from complications." This man likes to assure that his patients got the cold facts.

Kathy was devastated. I'd driven her to the appointment and when she got into the car she was depressed and crying. She had just been given a death sentence by a respected doctor. Who wouldn't be frantic?

"This is bull," I said. "You're young and you take care of yourself. There's no reason this should be so serious, so quickly!" I was furious at the unfeeling manner in which the doctor had treated her. "I'm taking you to an old friend of mine who's knowledgeable in environmental medicine. He treats difficult and unusual cases like this."

Alan Vinitsky, MD, is a certified specialist in internal medicine and pediatrics and had been studying alternative medical care and environmental- and allergy-related medical conditions for years. I knew Alan when I was a student at the dental school at the University of Pennsylvania and he was a student at the medical school.

The following week I took Kathy to Alan for a complete

workup, review and consultation. After evaluating all the data, and taking the *time* to *talk* and listen to her, Alan determined that she was suffering from mercury and arsenic poisoning. Symptoms of mercury toxicity can mimic many other disorders because the metal affects the enzyme synthesis and catalytic reactions in many body systems. It operates at a cellular level and can cause liver damage but also gastrointestinal disorders, thyroid dysfunction, skin and dermal reactions such as rashes, and neurological changes.

How could someone get that toxic from heavy metals in such a short time?

The apartment house in which she'd been living had an insect problem. To resolve the problem, the apartment management entered the affected apartments *weekly* and sprayed insecticide all around the rooms. They did the same thing throughout the building—stairwells, hallways, lobby—and all without the occupants' consent or knowledge. The spray was one of those odorless compounds that kill insects but were, of course, not concentrated enough to hurt *people*. She'd been inhaling this insecticide for months.

We also discovered that her hotel in Britain was built next to an old tannery that was no longer in business. Tanneries, as we've seen, used vast amounts of mercury in the processing of hides, with resulting effects on the workers similar to the hat manufacturers mentioned earlier. The tannery building and grounds were likely grossly contaminated with mercury, which was exposing people in the hotel to toxic vapors, worse while their windows were open.

It did not help that for most transatlantic airline flights, the cabins and overhead compartments are sprayed with an insecticide before the plane can leave to prevent unwanted insects from visiting and infesting another country. This was just another toxin Kathy was exposed to.

Alan Vinitsky treated Kathy for two years with various nutritional supplementation and chelation. The supplementation was needed to boost her physical health and enable her body to effectively fight her toxicity. The chelation was to find and remove as much mercury (and arsenic) from her body as possible.

Slowly, slowly she improved until eventually her normal health was restored.

ಎ

TROUBLES DOWN THE DRAIN

City codes require municipalities to remove mercury and other toxic metals from the public water supply, and the level of these metals in public water is also regulated in the United States by the Environmental Protection Agency. Although not officially acknowledged nationally, amalgam mercury fillings from dental offices result in enormous amounts of mercury being flushed into the water table or sewage systems and removing mercury from public water is extremely difficult. The California legislature has put it on record that "national studies and California studies show that the largest source of mercury in the wastewater comes from dental offices." Recognizing this at last, some communities are now passing legislation to prohibit dental dumping of mercury into the sewer lines.

For decades dentists have used basic "screen-type" filters for the vacuum systems at the dental chair. These traps are simple devices that catch only the largest pieces of mercury amalgam as they are removed from the tooth by the dentist and sucked out by the dental assistant. Periodically these traps are opened and the scrap mercury pieces are disposed of in a special toxic waste container, to be collected and recycled. The central vacuum unit itself, sitting in a closet or a basement, has its own covered canister, which catches mercury pieces and is also recycled periodically. But these devices do not adequately protect the public water supply and environment from mercury contaminationn, and clearly dentists should not be *adding* to the problem by placing new mercury amalgam fillings in

41

anyone's teeth. If they insist on doing so, they must use a less open precapsulated amalgam-alloy system. This method uses a premeasured amount of mercury in a closed mixing capsule with the alloy so liquid mercury vaporizes less in the ambient office air.

The Detroit Water and Sewerage Department has estimated that 10% to 15% of the dentists still placing these fillings are using raw liquid

> ...national studies and California studies show that the largest source of mercury in the wastewater comes from dental offices....
>
> *California Assembly Bill 611. Dental amalgam separators. Feb, 2003.*

mercury in their offices. Mercury in this form gives off the highest levels of vapor into the office environment. Who would want to breath this air for an hour or 2? For a whole career? These dentists are jeopardizing their own health and the health of their staff and their patients, while contaminating the wider environment in the process.

In 1984 the ADA's Council on Dental Materials, Instruments and Equipment recommended dentists discontinue use of bulk mercury and switch to the precapsulated amalgam systems. The ADA in 1994 and the Michigan Dental Association passed similar resolutions, again recommending non-use of bulk mercury by dentists. We must ask why some dentists so blatantly risk exposing themselves and others to this toxic metal.

And as the recognition of mercury's dangers increases and the reaction grows, all dentists must prevent contamination of the groundwater and waste water with the mercury released as old fillings are removed.

Amalgam separators are mercury-capture devices that can be installed in the main waste line of dental offices to remove most of the mercury "sludge" from waste water before it enters the community sewage system. The used and filled cannisters are sent to a company for environmental recycling. The International Standards Organization (ISO) developed a standard for these devices in 1999 (ISO 11143) and in 2003 the American Dental Association's board of trustees adopted mercury waste-handling and disposal standards for dental offices under their Best Management Practices (BMP). Yet most ADA members have still not installed these critical devices and the few who have installed them have done so because their local community or city ordinances require their use under penalty of law.

Years ago the Massachusetts Department of Environmental Protection determined the extreme level of contamination of waste water from dental offices with mercury from amalgam fillings. With the help of the Massachusetts Dental Society, they offered dentists in their state a voluntary compliance program to save them regulations and money by installing amalgam separators in their offices before March 1, 2005. After February 1, 2006 additional regulatory rules and fees would apply for mandatory amalgam separators to be installed. A large number of dentists appeared not to have complied with this request, even with incentives to clean up their act. It was necessary to legally require the separators be installed.

> In 1999, the International Standards Organization developed standards for amalgam separators.
>
> In 2003, the American Dental Association's board of trustees adopted mercury waste handling and disposal standards for dental offices.
>
> To date, most ADA members have not installed amalgam separators.

The San Francisco Bay Area Regional Water Quality Control Plant (RWQCP) has determined that amalgam separators installed in dental offices in the region would decrease mercury discharges into the air and water by 25% to 50%. California dentists were encouraged in 1996, in cooperation with the California Dental Association, to install separators to help clean up the waste water. In seven years only 7% of dentists complied and installed the devices. The California Assembly, in a bill introduced in 2003, stated that "voluntary means of compliance have not worked." Meanwhile Toronto, Ontario enacted an ordinance requiring dentists to install amalgam separators in their offices and one year later the amount of mercury going into the waste water declined by 58%.

MERCURY FILLINGS: HOW AND WHY

As we've seen, the original use of mercury goes back to the nineteenth century. There have only been minor changes in the actual techniques of placing a "silver" filling in a tooth that has been drilled and so has a hole in it. Briefly the current procedure, as still taught in dental schools as required by the ADA, is as follows.

The dental alloy is manufactured as a pellet of prepared solid metals supplied to the dentist in a closed plastic capsule. The alloy portion is mostly silver, usually with copper, tin and zinc added. The alloy pellet is on one side of a plastic divider and the liquid mercury is on the other side. When the tooth is ready to fill, the capsule is tightly squeezed end to end which pushes the mercury into the alloy. It is then put into a device, a miniature version of the machine the paint stores use to mix cans of paint, which quickly shakes it hard and for an exact period of time. Once mixed, the "amalgam" must be pushed into the tooth cavity within a certain period of time as the mix starts to set hard. The tooth cavity is filled up and the dentist carves the excess off so patients can put their teeth together when they bite.

The plastic capsule prevents any exposure or leakage of mercury or mercury vapor into the surroundings, until the alloy is mixed.

However as soon as the capsule is opened to release the mixed amalgam, mercury vapor floods the area and, unless protective measures are taken, is breathed in by everyone in the room. The vapor level will decrease after the amalgam "sets" hard but *it will continue to off-gas mercury vapor at high levels as long as it remains in the tooth.*

✿

Irene is a 35-year-old graphic artist. She'd returned to her regular dentist for a routine checkup. She had not had any decay for several years. When her dentist told her that she had a cavity that needed to be filled, she requested that a "non-silver" white filling be placed. The dentist completed the procedure and Irene returned home.

At home, she looked in the mirror and discovered to her horror that the new filling was silver colored and not white. The dentist had paid no attention to her request.

The next day at work she began to feel a tingling sensation down the outside of her right arm. This was the same side as the new silver filling. She was upset at being deceived and ignored. Luckily, the tingling sensation was temporary and disappeared in two weeks. She was uncomfortable for that time but she was able to work with the strange sensation in her arm.

✿

Dentists who think they're safe, who believe they are exposed to very little vapor, or who believe the ADA rhetoric about a safe level of mercury vapor, have not examined the evidence to the contrary. It's just common sense that the dentist and staff who are inhaling this mercury vapor all day are toxic with mercury in their systems. Even dentists who advertise that they do not place mercury fillings but only put in white bonded fillings are extensively exposed to mercury while taking out the old fillings. We're going to look at studies that reveal just how mercury toxic most dentists really are.

The ADA, the Schools and the Dentists

Every dental school in the country still teaches mercury amalgam fillings as a safe, proven method to fill cavities in teeth, and they most certainly fail to give their students a fair and balanced presentation of mercury use in dental fillings.[3]

Since the formation of the American Dental Association dentists have filled teeth with this alloy. When federal regulatory agencies came into being in the mid-twentieth century, it was common policy to grandfather in medical and dental procedures that had been used routinely up to that point. Any new procedure would have to undergo intense scrutiny by agencies like the US Environmental Protection Agency, the US Center for Disease Control or the US Food and Drug Administration. The primary mission of these watchdog agencies was to confirm that the new procedure would not harm any individual, make their health or medical condition worse, or cause them future injury. Unbiased safety studies are among the basic conditions a product, material or medicine must pass before it can be marketed to the public or professional community.

But dental amalgam fillings were grandfathered and therefore permitted without a standard safety review or classification. There are not and never have been any unbiased safety studies performed on dental amalgam. And the dental community, instead of reviewing the published scientific and toxicological studies and literature that has accrued over the last few decades, has avoided the issue. Their

---

[3] Since 1992, the Accreditation Council for Continuing Medical Education (ACCME®) has required that clinical recommendations be based on evidence accepted within the profession and that scientific research supporting recommendations meet generally accepted standards for experimental design, data collection, and analysis. (Source: ACCME CONTENT VALIDATION STATEMENT POLICY 2002-B-09) The American Medical Association requires that educational programs for healthcare professionals are scientifically based, accurate, current and objectively presented. (Source: American Medical Association Physician's Recognition Award Information Booklet for CME providers version 3.2)

policy: Don't ask. Don't tell.

This continued exposure of our population to mercury toxicity was allowed to continue officially until, as we'll see, September 7, 2006—Mercury Truth Day.

In many respects, the American Dental Association is more powerful than the US government, at least within its own niche. The ADA regulates and credentials all dental schools in the US. As part of that credentialing, *all American dental schools are required to teach the use of mercury amalgam fillings*. The failure of the dental schools to give a fair and balanced presentation of the facts parallels the ADA's selective dissemination of this vital information to their member dentists and the public. The ADA also indirectly controls all the state boards of dental examiners, who are usually members of the ADA. As part of this

There are not now and never have been any unbiased safety studies performed on dental amalgam. The dental community, instead of reviewing the published scientific and toxicological studies and literature that has accrued over the last few decades, has avoided the issue.

control, most of the boards of examiners of each state or region must include the placement of amalgam fillings as part of the dental board examinations. If the applicant does not wish to expose himself or his patient to mercury vapor, *he or she may not be able to pass the boards* and, of course, cannot get licensed. The fox has been set to guard the henhouse for a century. If dental students want to graduate dental school, they must expose themselves and their patients to mercury if they want to pass the program.

As if this were not astounding enough, since most of the members on the state boards of dentistry (which license the dentists in their states) are also members of the ADA, the ADA also has indirect control over the individuals who license dentists. For decades, local state licensing boards tried to silence dentists who told their patients the truth about the mercury in their fillings. Many dentists were persecuted and lost their licenses to practice because of this pressure to keep their mouths shut—effectively a gag order. In many cases, dentists have had to use their own money to defend themselves against a state-financed campaign to keep them from talking.

So why don't dentists take the initiative and do the investigating? Why don't they themselves evaluate the evidence, understand the need and change to safer, better fillings and tooth restorations? Because, as we've seen, change is hard.

Amalgam Fillings Up Close: Easy, not Pretty

At this time, mercury-amalgam fillings are still being used to fill cavities by about 50% of general dentists in the United States (and by many more dentists overseas). They use this alloy for the same reasons the American Society of Dental Surgeons was overthrown in the nineteenth century for not using it. Although its use is decreasing, mercury is still used for a host of reasons, most of which you won't like.

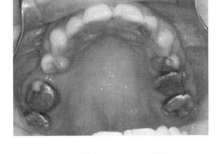

Figure 1-4: Old mercury fillings. Do they look safe and stable to you?

1. Mercury fillings are easy to use

The dentist or dental assistant simply takes a prepackaged plastic capsule out, squeezes it and puts it into a machine to thoroughly mix it. It is taken out of the capsule and transferred to the tooth a little at a time while the dentist packs it into the hole in the tooth. Excess is removed from the tooth surface and—voila!—the filling is in place. This procedure is so simple that dentists were able to train inexperienced staff to fill teeth before state laws forbade this practice.

This is in stark contrast to placing a modern white bonded resin into a tooth cavity. Bonded resins are very demanding and require precise technique if they are not to fail within a short time—one to two years sometimes. Sadly, some dentists find them too difficult to place and seem unable to place them with enough expertise or skill. A well bonded resin filling should last 10 to 20 years depending upon patient oral hygiene compliance and regular dental checkups.

2. Mercury fillings are fast

Prepackaged amalgam can be quickly compressed into the tooth. There are no absolute dry conditions to maintain as is necessary when placing a white bonded filling. In fact, zinc is put into the mercury alloy to *absorb* any moisture that gets into the alloy while it is setting.

3. Mercury fillings are cheap.

Mercury alloy is inexpensive for the dentist to purchase compared to bonded resin material. Resin fillings have many specific steps and several different components used in a specified order or the filling will not work (read decay quickly). Amalgam has only one.

Because they are fast to place, inexpensive and can be placed by any trained assistant, the dental office can place more fillings in less time (= more income). With auxiliary help, one dentist can treat more than one patient at a time.

4. Mercury fillings last several years before needing obvious replacement. See Figure 1-5, page 111.

Mercury amalgam alloy is a very hard material. After all, it is a metal alloy. As such it is not easily fractured and will stay in place until corroded or worn away, eventually fractured, or the tooth gives way by breaking or decaying—the most common reason. Even though amalgam fillings damage the tooth structure itself—we'll discuss later how damaging they are—and off-gas toxic vapor, it's usually a few years before the damage is visible and causes a major problem for the tooth—and you.

Being a hard material, they have been used to build up a tooth where a major part of the tooth structure has decayed or broken away. As a "build-up material," the remaining tooth is usually drilled down to a post-like shape so a full crown (cap) can be fabricated over it. For decades the material used for the cap has been a gold alloy, though unknown to the patient other metals are alloyed in the mix. (We'll look at that later too.)

For many patients, the contact between an amalgam filling and the metal of the cap on top of it—2 dissimilar metals—in the wet environment causes an electrical current to flow. This is called galvanic current—it's identical to the current generated by a battery—and can cause pain and destruction of the crowns and fillings themselves. Under these conditions, the mercury and other metals can leach out into the mouth at an accelerated rate, further increasing the potential toxic exposure of the patient (and breakdown of the filling).

5. Insurance companies pay a higher percentage towards mercury fillings; patients pay less out-of-pocket than for bonded resin fillings.

Let's face it—insurance companies like anything that saves them having to pay out from premiums collected. By continuing to pay a higher percentage for mercury-amalgam fillings, they can pay less total dollars than for bonded fillings that are safer but cost more.

Familiarity Breeds Content

Most dentists have become familiar and comfortable with things they learned in dental school years ago, things they still practice in their offices. When the first high-speed, water-cooled dental handpieces (drills) arrived, it took *years* for dentists to change their technique and begin using them. The evidence against the use of mercury dental fillings is available to any dentist who wishes to look. Most either do not want to know the truth because the truth would force them to change their procedures, or they're unable to admit that an older procedure, performed over decades, might actually be detrimental to their patients' health. They close their eyes to the facts or blindly follow whatever the American Dental Association recommends.

One of the major American manufacturers of the alloy that is mixed with mercury (in approximately 50:50 proportions) that produces and sells their product to dentists is Dispersalloy®. All products supplied to health practitioners that contain toxic or potentially toxic ingredients must legally come with a Material Safety Data Sheet (MSDS) as per the US Occupational Safety and Health Administration government guidelines. This form lists the ingredients of a product that are of questionable safety, what can be done for someone exposed to the substance and what *precautions the user must take when employing the product.*

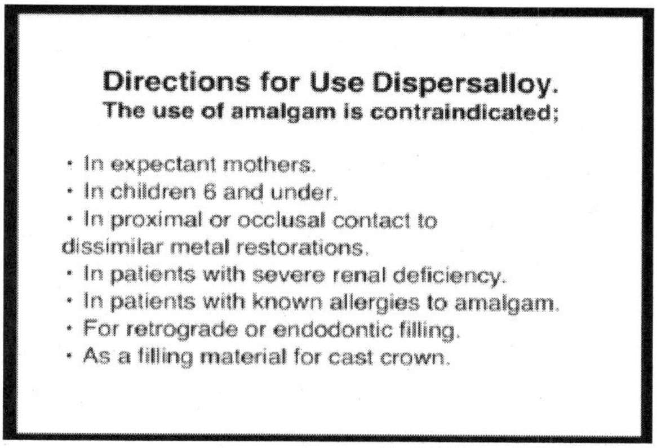

Figure 1-6 is a package insert supplied with Dispersalloy® to dentists. As you can see for yourself, every dentist who uses mercury alloy knows it is restricted in its use and

Directions for Use Dispersalloy.
The use of amalgam is contraindicated;

· In expectant mothers.
· In children 6 and under.
· In proximal or occlusal contact to dissimilar metal restorations.
· In patients with severe renal deficiency.
· In patients with known allergies to amalgam.
· For retrograde or endodontic filling.
· As a filling material for cast crown.

Figure 1-6: Package insert that comes with alloy for amalgam-mercury dental fillings

- ◆ cannot be used in pregnant mothers
- ◆ cannot be used in children under six years old
- ◆ cannot be used in contact with another metal in the next tooth
- ◆ cannot be used in people with kidney problems

Look at the label on the jar of dental amalgam filling material as it is supplied to the dentist (Figure 1-7). It clearly shows a skull and crossbones with the word "POISON" marked above it. There is a warning not to use it for children and it causes birth defects and other reproductive harm. Do you want this used in your mouth? The package insert is even scarier.

> The placement of…amalgam…will increase the level of mercury in the body of the patient.
>
> The health authorities of the various countries including Canada, Germany, France, The United Kingdom, Norway and Austria have recommended against placement…in …pregnant and nursing women and persons with impaired kidney function.

If a dentist tries to tell you it's okay to use mercury amalgam, ask him or her to show you the product insert. Then get out of that office as fast as you can.

I'm sorry to repeat this and I'm sorry if I must offend some of my professional colleagues, but most dentists do not think for themselves; they look to the ADA and do what the ADA says is acceptable. And therein lies the problem. Again, the American Dental Association, almost 150 years old, has never published an unbiased scientific article revealing the serious dangers of mercury vapor release from dental amalgam fillings to the patient, staff and doctor. I believe the ADA has, on the contrary, gone out of its way to find dentists and researchers who would support the pro-mercury filling position. Again this is not a "fair and balanced presentation." Valid and quite opposite scientific positions are not discussed in ADA articles, though such a policy is flatly contrary to medical education principles. The association successfully employed all its

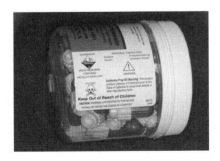

Figure 1-7: Mercury amalgam filling material supply jar with warnings on label

political might to sway government agencies to allow the continued use of mercury in patients' mouths. Until September 7, 2006.

September 7, 2006: Mercury Truth Day

For many years, groups of progressive, independent dentists, joined by activists, environmentalists, concerned mothers and other groups, have tried to get US government agencies to review the safety data (read "lack of safety data") on mercury dental fillings. Because of political pressure, mostly from the ADA, these agencies refused a hearing. It was only when the groups brought lawsuits against the agencies for not doing their job, for not protecting our population from harm, that any action began. It started at the grassroots level in various communities, with regulations by certain cities and states to manage the use of mercury and regulate dental-office use of mercury in the fillings. (See Appendix B, page 268, for a list of some of these new regulations and mandates listed by state and province.)

In 2006, the US Food and Drug Administration was challenged by a major coalition of groups—laypersons, environmentalists, scientists, medical and dental professionals and others—to examine scientific and medical evidence presented through published studies and testimony to determine if mercury dental fillings were neurotoxic to patients.

In September, 2006, the US FDA convened hearings in Maryland, with two independent panels of distinguished scientists addressing this issue. One panel consisted primarily of physicians, the other, primarily of dentists. Additional scientist-consultants were also on hand to testify. US FDA staff, supporting the ADA position on the total safety of mercury fillings, rolled out the same old rhetoric about mercury fillings being safe and stable. The studies presented were mostly old and their conclusions about mercury toxicity were even then misrepresented. The panels next heard testimony from expert witnesses who were able to demonstrate scientifically that mercury fillings pose a significant health risk. The independent panels voted 13 to seven to reject the US FDA staff position that mercury fillings are safe. The panels found that there was no basis for assuming the safety of mercury amalgam fillings. Not only could they not assure the public that mercury dental fillings were safe, but they recommended further study to determine how unsafe they may be.

> As of September 7, 2006, according to the US FDA, the use of mercury in dental fillings is unsafe.

In 1991, the World Health Organization confirmed that mercury contained in amalgam fillings is the greatest source of mercury vapor in non-industrialized settings, exposing the concerned population to mercury levels significantly exceeding those set for food and air.

Why Did It Take So Long?

The US FDA did not examine the safety of mercury fillings as it did that of drugs and medicines because, in the United States, amalgams were classified by the FDA as a "device" not a "substance". Under the US Code of Federal Regulations, amalgams were a prosthetic device:

> Amalgam Alloy, (a) Identification. An amalgam alloy is a device that consists of a metallic substance intended to be mixed with mercury to form filling material for treatment of dental caries.
> (b) Classification. Class II. (21 CFR 872.3050 (2001)

As a result of this classification, amalgams were never subject to official government testing in the United States, such as is required for medicines—until 2006. The US FDA maintains a web page on the use of amalgam, last updated in December 2002, on which it states, "No valid scientific evidence has shown that amalgams cause harm to patients with dental restorations, except in the rare case of allergy."

Even after September 2006, the US FDA failed to place amalgam filling material in a legal classification according to its safety in humans. It took a lawsuit by private parties (*Moms Against Mercury et al. v. Von Eschenbach, Commissioner, et al.*) that was not settled until May 2008. Through this suit, four nonprofit groups, two public officials, three dental professionals, and two consumer victims changed the US FDA's position. The US FDA website (http://www.fda.gov/cdrh/consumer/amalgams.html) now states:

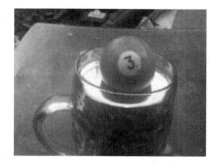

Figure 1-8: The FDA classified mercury amalgams as a device. Mercury is in fact a heavy metal and liquid at room temperature. Does a "device" appear to be holding up this billiard ball?

1. Dental amalgams contain mercury which may have neurotoxic effects on the nervous system of developing children and fetuses.
2. Amalgam fillings release mercury vapor in the mouth, during placement, removal and chewing.

The revolution has begun!

MERCURY AND OUR BODIES

The basic composition of dental amalgam hasn't changed much since the nineteenth century. As previously stated, the filling material is composed of roughly 50% elemental mercury and the other 50% is mostly silver with tin, zinc and copper added to help the alloy handle and behave better. This mixture of metals is left in a liquid, acidic environment—the mouth. Just as our metal lawn furniture, left out in the rain, oxidizes and corrodes, the alloy breaks down and loses metal atoms as it rusts. Even under crowns, the mercury leaches out through the root into the surrounding osseous tissues and blood vessels.

There are two serious problems with mercury-amalgam fillings: this leaching and off-gassing of mercury, copper and tin, and the fact that the amalgam fillings corrode and expand inside the tooth. We are going to look at each of these dangers in detail.

Amalgam Problems 1: Off-gassing and Leaching of Toxic Metal

Dental amalgam fillings are not stable. They release mercury vapor into the mouth continuously from the day they're placed in the tooth to the day they're removed. Tin[4] and copper are also released and excessive absorption of those two metals can also cause negative health consequences (see Wilson's Disease[5]), though they are not as toxic as mercury.

The mercury is released as an inorganic elemental vapor and 75% to 80% of that vapor is inhaled into the lungs. It can also be absorbed through the oral soft tissues (as it can through the skin) or swallowed accidentally. From the lungs, it immediately enters the blood stream and is converted within minutes to methylmercury, an organic, fat-soluble form of mercury. These molecules are then deposited in the body's fat reserves and liver. That is why a simple blood test will not show mercury toxicity: mercury is not present in the blood for more than minutes. If it's not in the blood, it won't be excreted in

---

[4] Tin excesses can be from dental fillings, stannous fluoride in toothpastes or water exposed to brass- or tin-containing solders. The organic forms of tin are more toxic and are commonly from herbicide, insecticides or fungicides. Tin can cause headaches (cerebral edema) and suppression of the immune system.

[5] Wilson's disease is caused by excess copper in the body's tissues with inherent increases in urinary copper excretion. The condition which can be genetic in origin, can also be caused by absorption of copper from water pipes, made worse with the water chlorination process. Symptoms are indicative of liver dysfunction with neurological and blood abnormalities.

the urine. If your doctor rules out mercury toxicity or poisoning in your body by ordering a simple urine or blood test, he does not know how to evaluate heavy-metal exposure. Those tests will usually come back negative and he will report that you are not metal toxic. But you may be.

Human studies show that dental amalgam contributes significantly to mercury body burden in humans who have amalgam fillings.

How much mercury is released by a dental amalgam depends on how large the filling is. But studies have shown that

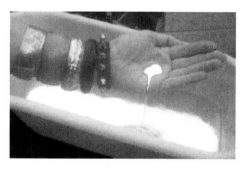

Figure 1-9: This is not recommended. Toxic mercury is absorbed through the skin.

an amalgam filling with an average surface area of 40 square millimeters (about 6 mm × 6 mm)—about the size of a one surface molar filling—will give off 15 micrograms of mercury vapor per day. Figure 1-10, page 111 shows an old 2-surface amalgam filling of approximately 90 square millimeters. This filling gives off about 32 micrograms of mercury per day through mechanical wear and evaporation and dissolution in saliva. Other studies have found 12 or fewer filling surfaces release 29 micrograms of mercury per day, while four or fewer filling surfaces released 8 micrograms. My own clinical study (over 1500 cases) shows patients with more than two or three amalgam fillings release oral mercury vapor in excess of the maximum limits the US EPA sets for increased health risks.

In a study published in the dental journal *Dental Materials* in 1994, a mercury amalgam used by dentists was soaked in various solutions. The results were solutions rendered severely cytotoxic—that is, able to kill cells—by the mercury that had leaked out of the filling material.

So there is no question: mercury is absorbed into your body constantly from dental fillings. The body is also exposed to the mercury released from under some crowns. See Figure 1-5, page 111. This is no small amount of toxic metal, with one study showing 101 milligrams of mercury released into the mouth from under a single gold crown over a period of nine years.

※

She kind of looked like a typical grandmother: slightly frizzy, faded grayish-brown hair held in place with a clip and no make-up. Joan was a smallish woman, about five foot four inches, wearing a light-colored shirt with pastel stripes and beige slacks. At 65 years of age, she had a younger, livelier attitude than one might have expected.

But she wasn't happy. When I began questioning her during the biologic dental consultation, the whole story came out.

"We were going to visit Africa. My husband always wanted to go on a safari and this was our chance. We wanted to see the animals in their natural habitat. So we went to our physician and he told us we needed to get several vaccinations. Yellow fever, Danang fever or something like that. So we got three vaccinations that day. It was about a month before the trip. That was when the trouble started. Just me—my husband was fine.

"A little over one week after the injections I got burning and pain down both my arms. My fingertips seemed somehow numb and burning at the same time. And my one shoulder ached. Our doctor didn't know what to do. I went to a couple of others and was told the pain and tingling were from the mercury in the vaccinations. I was toxic from the injections and would need to have treatment, chelation he called it, to get the mercury out of my body. But it couldn't be started until after we got back from our trip. It nearly ruined the vacation having the pain in my arms."

She was rubbing her arms absent-mindedly.

"How long ago was your trip?" I asked.

"We got back three months ago. I wanted to start the treatments immediately but the doctor said I needed to see you first because of my mercury dental fillings."

Her doctor was right.

"Joan, the mercury in your dental fillings constantly gives off mercury vapor into your body. There's no point in chelating your body to remove imbedded and absorbed mercury if your teeth are going to re-contaminate you immediately. Once the fillings are safely replaced you can begin chelating the mercury out of your body tissues. Hopefully the changes in your arms will reverse and you will feel normal again."

Joan's oral mercury vapor readings when we began were 11.0 micrograms per cubic meter resting. After chewing for three minutes her mercury level went up to 59 micrograms per cubic meter. She had 17 surfaces of mercury dental fillings in her teeth. As you'll soon read, these readings are six times the safe health level set by the US Environmental Protection Agency, which is 9 micrograms per cubic meter adjusted.

We removed her amalgam fillings, replacing them with bonded restorations over three months. Because of her toxic reaction to the vaccines, it was necessary to go beyond our basic safety protocol while removing her fillings. To safeguard against Joan having additional toxic changes from any incidental mercury absorption while we were drilling out the fillings, we sent her straight to her physician after each dental visit and he administered an intravenous flush with vitamin C and glutathione. Those chelating agents helped her body remove the mercury before more was absorbed into her tissues.

After all the mercury amalgams were replaced, we tested Joan for oral mercury vapor again. Her readings four months later were down to 0.0 at her resting level and 1.3 after chewing. The additional exposure to mercury from her dental fillings was gone.

However, I'm sorry to report that one year after beginning chelation treatment with her physician to remove the mercury in her body, Joan was still in pain with tingling still in her arms. Although early reversal of mercury exposure may restore pre-exposure health, in some cases the physical damage caused by the mercury killing cells and nerve tissue is not reversible. Remember the Mad Hatter's neurological disease and my reference to Alzheimer's disease.

Although mercury in vaccinations (as the preservative thimerosal) has been all but removed from pediatric vaccines, as noted earlier, *all adult vaccines still contain this toxic chemical.* Unfortunately Joan was susceptible to the thimerosal and her body reacted badly to its exposure. In my opinion, if a vaccination containing thimerosal is needed, vitamin and detoxifying supplementation is needed prior to the injection to protect the body from absorbing the mercury that is injected. There are ways to supplement the body's defenses against heavy metals and protect against additional toxic effects of the mercury. Homeopathic remedies are sometimes very effective in chelating or removing heavy metals from the body.

I treat several patients each month who have been referred to me by physicians and other healthcare professionals who are able to recognize heavy metal toxicity. They know that the mercury in their patients' teeth must be removed before general chelation to remove the body burden of mercury can begin. If patients are severely health compromised and debilitated, I recommend that on the day mercury filings are removed they immediately see their physician for intravenous chelation with vitamin C, glutathione or DMSA. This is to prevent any mercury that might have been absorbed during the fillings' removal from staying in the body and making the patient yet more toxic and more ill.

Measuring Mercury Vapor in the Mouth

The concentration of mercury vapor in the mouth can be accurately measured, directly in the mouth. In my practice we have a device called an atomic absorption spectrometer. Our model is the

Hg253 Portable Mercury Analyzer (Genesis Laboratory Systems, Inc., Grand Junction, Colo). (See Figure 1-11.) There are other analytical devices to measure mercury vapor levels but the atomic spectrometer actually measures mercury atoms and is therefore more accurate.

Since 2003, we have been conducting an ongoing study of my patients by recording their oral mercury vapor levels. This measurement objectively demonstrates the off-gassing of mercury vapor from the mercury amalgam fillings.

All my new patients, and my existing patients, as they come in for their 6-month checkups, are tested for their oral mercury vapor levels. The process only takes a few minutes and is painless. The results surprise a lot of people who have been told for years that there is no risk from dental amalgam fillings. It motivates them to take action and protect their bodies from further mercury exposure. Our testing procedure is as follows;

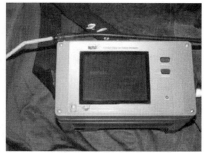

1. The date, patient's name, age are recorded on a special form. (See Figure 1-14.)

Figure 1-11: Portable Mercury Vapor Analyzer (Genesis Laboratory Systems, Inc.)

2. The patient is asked if they have eaten any large type of fish, such as tuna, marlin or swordfish, in the previous week. If so, how many times and when.

3. The number of amalgam filling surfaces in the teeth is recorded.

4. A reading of the room mercury vapor level is taken to assure there is no vapor from the room to affect the patient's reading.

5. Before any procedures are done in the mouth, an initial reading of the patient's resting oral vapor level is taken. The device samples the oral air with a plastic straw which is held in the mouth

above the tooth surfaces. The unit samples the air, displaying the mercury vapor levels on the display continuously. The highest reading displayed is recorded as the patient's resting oral mercury vapor level in micrograms of vapor-phase elemental mercury per cubic meter. (See Figures 1-12 and 1-13.)

6. The patient is then asked to chew sugarless gum for three minutes. At the end of that time another reading is taken.

7. The readings are recorded on a special form, a copy is given to the patient and the results are then discussed with the patient.

A person's resting level of mercury vapor recorded is present in their mouth 24 hours a day, seven days a week. If he or she stimulates the surface of the filling by, say, chewing, the metal reacts as you would expect: the number of released molecules increases just as boiling water increases the release of water molecules as steam. This stimulation can occur when

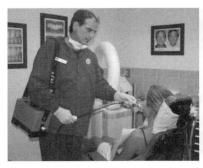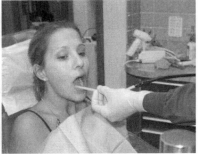

Figures 1-12 and 1-13: Taking an oral mercury vapor level reading

♦ Chewing, with or without food
♦ Drinking hot beverages like tea or coffee
♦ Drinking acidic drinks like lemonade, limeade or sodas
♦ Getting your teeth polished at the dentist office, a procedure that heats and abrades the filling surfaces.

The vapor level after these actions can increase 10 to 100 times or more over their resting level of mercury.

You'll see from this sample test form (Figure 1-14) that the room mercury vapor level was zero. This patient has six mercury amalgam fillings in his teeth. This does not mean six teeth because one tooth can have up to five of its sides filled with amalgam. Initial testing at rest revealed a vapor level of 59.3 micrograms per cubic meter (m³) of air. This is high and indicates a large amount of mercury coming off the six surfaces of fillings. The US maximum allowable levels of

---

Dental Learning Resource, LLC
DONALD ROBBINS, DMD, FAGD, IAOMT
Safe Biologic Dentistry

(2)

DATE: _2/07/07_   NAME: ▮▮▮▮▮▮▮▮   AGE: _36_

Room Reading ___0.0___ microg/m³

YOUR ORAL HG VAPOR LEVEL IS _59.3_ **microg/m³**

For 24hrs/7days/wk

After heat or chewing your level is _129.9_ microg/m³

Large Fish consumed over last week: ___None___

You have # _6_ mercury/silver filling surfaces in your mouth

EPA: MAXIMUM INHALATION LEVEL BEFORE TOXIC SYMPTOMS:
8 mmg/cm³

Mercury vapor is **continually** being released from the mercury fillings. The amount of mercury released and absorbed by your body depends on how many fillings you have and how old they are.

MAXIMUM PERMISSIBLE INDUSTRIAL MERCURY EXPOSURE
LEVEL (for American workers with protection) IS:

1) American Conference of Governmental Industrial Hygienists (ACGIH) — **25 mmg/m³** for 8hr/day/5 day week
2) National Institute for Occupational Safety and Health (NIOSH) — **50 mmg/m³** for 10hr/day/4 day week
3) Occupational Safety and Health Administration [Final Rule Limit] (OSHA) — **100 mmg/m³** for 8hr/day/5 day week

Additional information can be obtained online at:

1. www.iaomt.org
2. www.toxicteeth.org
3. www.abcmt.com
4. www.momsagainstmercury.org
5. www.generationrescue.org

FOR FLUORIDE DANGERS:
1. www.fluoridealert.org/
2. www.FluorideAction.Net
3. www.orgsites.com/ny/nyscof

340 North Route 100 (Across from Target) | P.O. Box 449 | Exton, PA 19341
Phone: 610.363.1980 | Fax: 610.363.7798 | www.dentallearningresource.com

Figure 1-14: A mercury vapor test form used in my office.

mercury-vapor exposure, the highest allowed for an *industrial worker*, is 100 micrograms per cubic meter over a 40-hour work week (OSHA). (See the section below for the maximum vapor limits allowed by the US government and some state agencies.) But that allowable limit is for a 40-hour exposure in a 7-day week. This patient's 59.3 reading is constant for a 168 hour full week (24 hours per day × seven days) which is four times the exposure of a 40-hour work week. Thus the patient's mercury reading at rest in my office was *more than 2½ times the* highest *industrial federal limit*.

After chewing for three minutes his level went up to 129.9 micrograms per cubic meter. This is not constant all day but it does require about 1½ hours for the elevated level to go back down to the resting level, assuming no further activation of the surface of the fillings. Note that 129.9 micrograms per cubic meter is 1.3 times the 100 micrograms per cubic meter maximum rate of exposure allowed by OSHA ($^{129.9}/_{100}$ = 1.3). Also, if this exposure continued all day (for example chewing gum), the exposure would not be just a 40 hour work week. It would be 4.2 times the maximum work week (168 hours per week/40 hour work = 4.2). Therefore my patient's cumulative exposure is over *five times the Federal maximum limit of industrial mercury vapor exposure*.

And if we consider this is actually a non-industrial reading and is meant to apply to the general population in a *residential setting*, the inhalation level allowed, according to the EPA, must be less than 9 microgram per cubic meter, not 100 microgram per cubic meter. We do our calculation like this: five times the industrial level of 100 micrograms per cubic meter divided by the 9 microgram per cubic meter inhalation level allowed by the US EPA ($5 \times {}^{100}/_{9}$). So for individual inhalation exposures, the "5 times acceptable level" turns out to be *fifty times the maximum* allowed outside an industrial-work setting.

Where does the mercury go? As we saw, it's inhaled into the lungs, absorbed into the blood stream and converted almost immediately to methylmercury, the organic form of mercury, most dangerous to our health. If this patient's body cannot efficiently excrete the mercury, he will show some evidence of poor health or sickness, either in the short term (days or weeks) or long term (years with chronic exposure).

Mercury Vapor Study Results

In 2004 I began to keep careful records of the levels of mercury vapor in my patients' mouths.[6] My analysis of the results I obtained from testing over 1,200 patients has turned up some significant evidence.

1. The more surfaces of amalgam fillings a person has, the more mercury vapor is given off into the mouth.

2. Eating fish has little if no effect on the level of mercury vapor in the mouth.

3. Activation of the surface of mercury amalgam dental fillings by

+ chewing, with or without food
+ drinking hot beverages like coffee or tea
+ eating or drinking acidic foods like lemonade
+ carbonated beverages like sodas

will increase the amount of mercury vapor releasing from the filling surface.

4. If amalgam fillings are safely removed from the mouth (replaced with non-metallic bonded restorations), the level of mercury vapor drops proportionately.

5. If all the amalgam fillings are removed from the mouth, the

---

[6] The data I used to generate graphs 1-2, 1-3 and 1-4 were collected and evaluated statistically. Parameters that could influence data readings include volume of amalgam filling (not just surfaces), variations in mercury content of each filling (usually determined from the original mixed ratio of mercury to alloy), soft tissue interference with a sampling wand (puffy cheeks, large tongue, facial structure), breathing patterns. I am preparing these data for scientific publication.

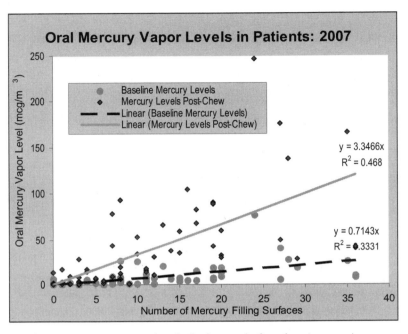

Graph 1-2: Mercury vapor levels (before and after chewing gum) correlate with the number of mercury amalgam fillings surfaces present in my patients' mouths.

patient's oral mercury vapor levels go to 0 or very close to 0.

I've assembled the data I collected during the year prior to writing this book and used it to construct three graphs. This is what they show: Graph 1-2 shows the number of mercury amalgam fillings ranged from 0 to 36 surfaces. Before chewing gum activated the filling surfaces, mercury vapor levels ranged from 0 to 76.3 micrograms per cubic meter. Note the dashed line showing the increase in vapor levels as the number of fillings increases. After chewing activated the filling surfaces, the mercury vapor levels ranged from 0 to 246.8 micrograms per cubic meter, also increasing as the number of fillings increases (the solid grey line).

This is clear evidence of a pattern: the more mercury amalgam

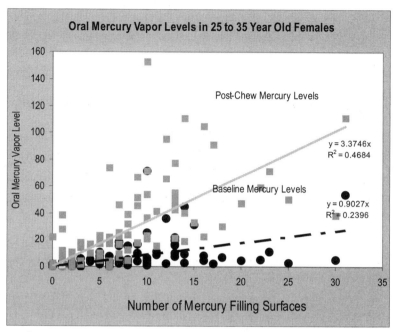

Graph 1-3; Mercury levels measured in women aged 25 to 35 correlate with the number of amalgam filling surfaces present in their mouths.

fillings in a person's teeth, the higher the mercury vapor levels in the mouth, which leads to more toxic mercury absorption in the body.

Graph 1-3 preliminary results demonstrate a strong correlation: for these woman of child-bearing age: more mercury fillings in their teeth result in a higher mercury exposure. This line chart shows a strong correlation to Graph 1-2 which shows results from the overall population. For women who are pregnant or nursing, mercury absorbed could accumulate in the fetus or nursing baby at a rate far higher than the accumulation rate in the mother.

Maximum Allowable Mercury Levels

It is now widely accepted that *there is no safe limit* and almost any amount of mercury can have negative health consequences. It is also

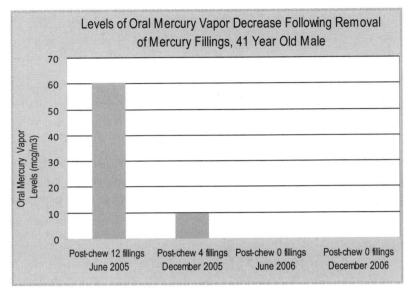

Graph 1-4: Mercury vapor levels measured before and after mercury fillings were removed from the teeth of a 41-year-old male patient. The sampling took place over approximately 1½ years, during which the patient had all his mercury-malgam fillings replaced with bonded resin fillings. His oral mercury exposure dropped with each section of mercury removal. This example of reduced exposure following dental filling removal is representative of most of the patients I've treated. Note that the zero mercury reading continued six months after the first clean reading with no dental amalgam fillings left. When amalgam fillings are removed, the reduction in mercury exposure appears to be permanent.

generally agreed that inhaled mercury vapor is the most toxic form likely to be experienced by the average person. Nonetheless, government oversight agencies have attempted in the past to establish a "safe" level of mercury exposure. In each case exposure above the listed level results in the appearance of adverse health effects.

♦ The US Occupational Safety and Hazard Administration (OSHA) set their occupational worker safety levels at 100 micrograms per cubic meter for a 40-hour work week. (Some published standards for OSHA list 50 micrograms per cubic meter as the acceptable level.[7]) If a worker is exposed to that concentration of mercury vapor in less time, they are not allowed to work additional hours that whole week.

♦ The National Institute for Occupational Safety and Health (NIOSH) has set its time-weighted average (TWA)[8] threshold-limit value of 50 micrograms per cubic meter. The NIOSH limit is based on the risk of central nervous system damage and eye, skin, and respiratory tract irritation [NIOSH 1992].

♦ The American Conference of Governmental Industrial Hygienists (ACGIH) assigned a threshold limit value (TLV)[9] of 25 micrograms per cubic meter for an eight-hour workday or 40-hour workweek exposure.

♦ The US Environmental Protection Agency (EPA) sets their lowest observable adverse effect level (LOAEL) at 25 micrograms per cubic meter. Above this level hand tremors, increased memory disturbances, and autonomic nervous system disorders (for example heart rate, sweating, breathing regularity) appeared. However when evaluated by the allowed *inhalation* level of mercury vapor, the EPA only allows 9 micrograms per cubic meter.

♦ The US Agency for Toxic Substances and Disease Registry (ATSDR) of the CDC has set the minimal risk levels (MRL) for *inhaled* mercury at 0.2 micrograms per cubic meter, a very low level indeed.

♦ Some studies show lower TWAs of 25 to 40 micrograms per cubic meter.

♦ Health Canada, in a final report by the Environmental Health Directorate, has called for the elimination of mercury dental fillings and

---

[7] EPA report, January 2007: Mercury, elemental (CASRN 7439-97-6) IRIS Substance.

[8] TWA or time-weighted average is the "allowable" exposure concentration over a normal 8-hour workday or a 40-hour work week. Above this level the studies reviewed by the organization showed adverse health effects appearing.

[9] TLV or threshold limit value is the concentration to which workers can be exposed without adverse health effects.

has established the tolerable daily intake (TDI) of mercury vapor at 1 microgram per day.

Mercury Exposure: the Bottom Line

The whole question of what exposure level will cause symptoms of toxicity is a vexing one. There are generally three levels of public exposure to mercury vapor:

Industrial Level (50-100 micrograms per cubic meter). US Occupational Safety and Health Administration (OSHA) levels of "acceptable" mercury vapor exposure are the highest allowable. They are based on workers in hostile environments that use extreme ventilation systems and other technologies to move contaminated air out of the workplace quickly. Because of those working practices, mercury concentrations are set higher than other situations because hopefully the vapor is dissipated quickly enough that workers do not inhale or absorb toxic levels of mercury. Also, workers' exposure is limited to the 40-hour work week.

Non-Residential Level (3-10 micrograms per cubic meter). Over 10 micrograms is the cutoff point. Anything more than that and the item contaminated with mercury should be disposed of. Over 3 micrograms requires vacating the buildings until remedial efforts lower the concentration exposure. These levels are lower than 10 micrograms for day care centers, schools, stores and malls, churches, etc.

Residential Level (0.3-3 micrograms per cubic meter). Because residential sites are not designed with large and efficient air circulators and fans, it is important to limit the level of an acceptable mercury vapor exposure. Below this level unwanted health effects are not expected to appear, even in children and pregnant women. The EPA and the Agency ffor Toxic Substance and Disease Registry (ATSDR) both accept 0.3 micrograms as the maximum level of mercury vapor exposure for safe occupation of a home or residence.

A True Story

⟪@

For many years a company in Gloucester County, New Jersey manufactured thermometers and other mercury-containing devices on a site in Franklin Township. In June, 1984, the site was purchased by the Accutherm company to produce thermometers.

In November, 1987, Accutherm was notified by the Gloucester County Health Department that there was a high level of tetrachloroethylene (a carcinogen) in the drinking water of the surrounding area. This contamination was traced back to the Accutherm site. By mid-1988 the New Jersey Department of Environmental Protection (NJDEP) and the Occupational Safety and Hazard Administration (OSHA) had determined the site was contaminated with mercury and petroleum hydrocarbons as well, and the company septic system was contaminating the surrounding area.

Nothing was apparently done for some time about cleaning up the contamination. In 1994 when Accutherm ceased operations. Inspections revealed mercury vapor was present at over three times OSHA allowable levels. Visible liquid mercury was seen on the site in the floorboards. The NJDEP kept sending notices to Accutherm requiring cleanup of the site and posting of hazard notices. Again, no action was accomplished. In 1995, the United States Environmental Protection Agency (US EPA) assessed the property. Their report read that "...the site does not present an immediate threat to human health or the environment." They did observe "several small droplets of Hg were located on the floor..." as were various mercury devices and vials.

The site was legally transferred to Navillus Group, LLC on the basis of the US EPA's older assessment that the site did not require a removal action and further study was indicated (1996). Navillus proceeded to rehabilitate the building in 2002 and a partner, Jim Sullivan, Inc., purchased it outright for use as a daycare center. After several approvals had been granted by the Franklin Township authorities, the daycare facility, Kiddie Kollege, was approved in February 11, 2004 and began to admit children.

In April 2006, the New Jersey Department of Environmental Protection (NJDEP) required the owner to have analyses performed to demonstrate that contaminant levels were below acceptable standards. On July 28, 2006, the NJDEP received test results of the indoor mercury levels, levels so high that the building was declared unfit for occupancy. Local officials and the owner and tenant were notified the building was not to be used or inhabited until further notice.

Further inspection revealed metallic mercury droplets in the basement and between the floor joists of the building. The drinking water, from private wells, also appeared contaminated.

It took almost 20 years to close down this contaminated toxic site. Meanwhile almost 100 children—some as young as eight months of age—had gone through the daycare and had been exposed to poisonous mercury vapor. The owner of the daycare was pregnant and exposed for long periods of time without knowing it. As reported by Jan Hefler, a *Philadelphia Inquirer* reporter, as long as seven weeks after the daycare closed, over a dozen children still had elevated levels of mercury in their bodies and one 5-year-old girl still had seizures, rashes and peeling skin on her fingers and toes.

What is the point of this story?

The NJDEP went into the building during the assessment wearing hazmat suits and portable mercury-vapor measuring devices similar to the unit I use in my practice to measure oral mercury vapor levels. The readings they got in the room occupied by the children were high enough for them to declare the building uninhabitable and shut it down. Those readings were *7.0 and 8.4 micrograms per cubic meter.* As we've seen, *most of my patients who have more than a couple of mercury amalgam fillings show readings well in excess of those numbers.*

❧

Measuring Mercury Levels in the Body

We're all familiar with the old adage, if all you have is a hammer, everything looks like a nail. If a doctor has only one type of treatment to offer patients, he or she may miss the diagnosis of conditions requiring a different treatment. Many doctors have not been trained sufficiently in recognizing and treating patients suffering from heavy metal toxicity and are not aware of the myriad of symptoms that affect many body systems that may look like a typical disease. A good diagnostic physician will consider all the possibilities that may cause a patient's symptoms and rule them out one by one until the ultimate cause is found.

A few pages back, I told the story of Joan, whose system was contaminated with high levels of mercury. Yet running a simple urine or blood test on Joan would not have shown any mercury levels in her body. Her high body burden of mercury was not actively circulating in her blood. A different type of test is required. Two of the more common tests are the urine challenge test and the fecal challenge test.

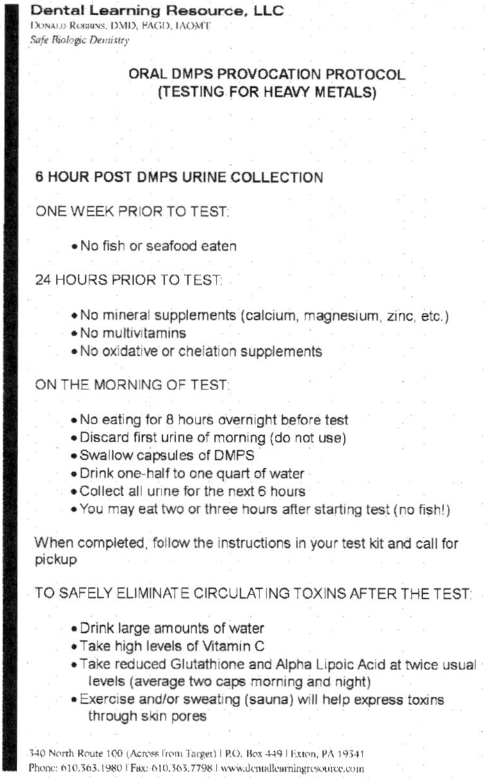

Dental Learning Resource, LLC
Donald Robbins, DMD, FAGD, IAOMT
Safe Biologic Dentistry

ORAL DMPS PROVOCATION PROTOCOL
(TESTING FOR HEAVY METALS)

6 HOUR POST DMPS URINE COLLECTION

ONE WEEK PRIOR TO TEST:

• No fish or seafood eaten

24 HOURS PRIOR TO TEST:

• No mineral supplements (calcium, magnesium, zinc, etc.)
• No multivitamins
• No oxidative or chelation supplements

ON THE MORNING OF TEST:

• No eating for 8 hours overnight before test
• Discard first urine of morning (do not use)
• Swallow capsules of DMPS
• Drink one-half to one quart of water
• Collect all urine for the next 6 hours
• You may eat two or three hours after starting test (no fish!)

When completed, follow the instructions in your test kit and call for pickup

TO SAFELY ELIMINATE CIRCULATING TOXINS AFTER THE TEST:

• Drink large amounts of water
• Take high levels of Vitamin C
• Take reduced Glutathione and Alpha Lipoic Acid at twice usual levels (average two caps morning and night)
• Exercise and/or sweating (sauna) will help express toxins through skin pores

340 North Route 100 (Across from Target) | P.O. Box 449 | Exton, PA 19341
Phone: 610.363.1980 | Fax: 610.363.7798 | www.dentallearningresource.com

Figure 1-15: Instruction sheet for DMPS provocation urine test

The Urine Challenge Test

A urine challenge test measures urinary mercury levels after oral 2,3-dimercaptopropane-1-sulfonate (DMPS) or oral meso-2, 3-dimercaptosuccinic acid (DMSA) administration. These are provoking chemical agents that primarily mobilize the fat stores in the patient's body. This mobilization gives the clinician a picture of the level of toxic metals in the body tissues. This test is a better indicator of the mercury stored in fat tissue and the overall mercury burden of the liver and kidneys than a test performed without the challenging agent. This is the test my office usually orders (with physician approval) if patients have not been tested in this manner previously and are not in a debilitated condition. There is a pre-test protocol (Figure 1-15) that patients follow before taking the test. They consume no fish or seafood for one week prior and must refrain from using any detoxifying or chelating supplements, including vitamin C, alpha lipoic acid, reduced glutathione and selenium for 24 hours before the test. Patients void their first urine in the morning. They then swallow a capsule(s) of a chemical agent, DMPS or DMSA, with a full glass of water and collect their urine for

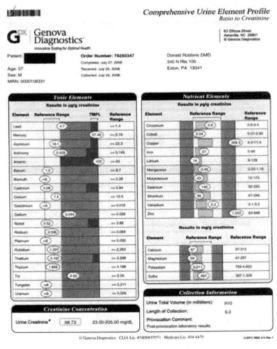

Figure 1-16: Sample post provocation urine test result

six hours, sometimes 24 hours. The sample is sent to the diagnostic laboratory via mail express and the test results are sent to the doctor's office, usually within one week.

Figure 1-16 shows an example of test results for an actual patient. In this sample report you can see that 20 toxic elements are measured and 15 nutrient element levels are reported. This patient had serious toxic levels of mercury and arsenic. There was elevation of their tin and gallium levels. The copper level was also too high, even though a small amount of copper is needed in the body for normal function. Excessive zinc is usually not a serious problem.

The Fecal Challenge Test

Similar to the urine challenge test, the fecal challenge test shows toxic metals being excreted from the body. (See Figure 1-17.) The pre-test protocol and the challenge chemical agents are similar to those for the urine test. A stool sample must be collected and sent to the diagnostic laboratory.

Some doctors routinely order a hair analysis test. This is often done on a young child where compliance with the other two tests is not dependable. In this test a small amount of hair is

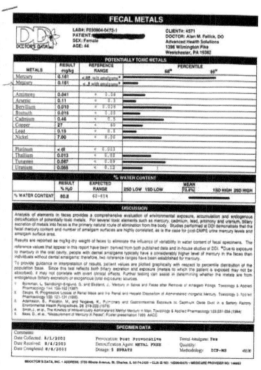

Fiigure 1-17: Sample post provocation fecal test result

cut off the patient and sent to a laboratory for analysis of mercury content. However, in my opinion the hair analysis test is almost diagnostically useless because, if the hair comes back negative for mercury, it can mean two quite opposite things. Either the patient has no mercury in their body or they cannot excrete mercury that is present in their body. On the other hand, if the hair comes back positive for mercury it means the patient is capable of excreting mercury. It does not tell you if the amount of mercury in the body is tiny or seriously high. Knowing the patient can excrete mercury does not tell the doctor if or how they can be treated, or even if they need chelation to remove a body burden of mercury.

The Baddest Tattoo

The familiar ornamental tattoo requires the deposition of silver salts into the skin to leave a permanent image or "marker." Dentistry offers mankind something called an "amalgam tattoo."

Amalgam fillings, as we've seen, have silver as one of their components. If the dentist is not careful when putting an amalgam into a tooth cavity, he can inadvertently push the alloy into the mucosal tissues. The mucosa is the soft tissue lining of the mouth. This poor technique leaves a permanent black silver-mercury residue in the tissues that is much like a tattoo on the skin. (See Figure 1-18, page 111.) Mercury may also leach out from the tooth filling slowly into the overlying gum tissue. We see this with large amalgam fillings placed well beneath the height of the gingiva, which is the attached gum around the teeth.

These imbedded mercury-silver tattoos have been ignored by organized dentistry since amalgam fillings were first used. This is a huge mistake because the mercury in this sort of tattoo is in *direct contact with oral tissues, blood vessels and nerves.* The material is *still leaching out mercury, but now directly into the patient's body tissues.* There is an exceptionally high concentration of mercury in these contaminated tissues, with estimates as high as 380 micrograms of mercury per gram of tissue. Compare that to the concentration of mercury in gum tissues when not in direct contact with the amalgam fillings: 2.3 micrograms mercury per gram of tissue.

This is a gross exposure to a dangerous substance and the tattoo *must be removed surgically.* The excised tissue is usually sent to oral pathology for a biopsy report. A sample report is shown in Figure 1-19.

Most dentists don't realize there's danger in these tattoos. Yet

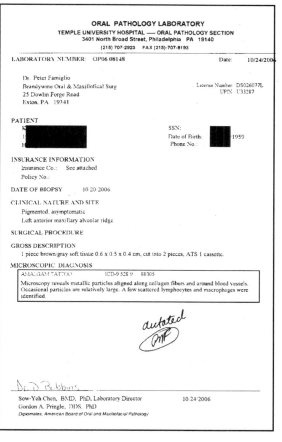

Figure 1-19: Amalgam tattoo pathology report

look at the pathologist's microscopic analysis and diagnosis. There are *"metallic particles…around blood vessels."* The lymphocytes and macrophages are involved. These cells are activated to fight invasion of the body by foreign substances. *This is a continuous and chronic inflammatory response that will not end until the substance is gone.* The level of mercury exposure from these imbedded particles is enormous. The constant effort by the body to remove these toxic materials can fatigue the strongest immune systems.

A 1995 study of lichen planus, a mucosal tissue change thought to be precancerous, showed that removal of mercury amalgam fillings resolved the symptoms in most of the patients with this condition.

AMALGAM PROBLEMS II: CORROSION AND EXPANSION OF THE FILLINGS

When I was in dental school we were taught mercury amalgams were safe and they were the best restorative material to put in a back tooth (a molar). This is a blatant lie still being taught in almost every dental school in the country. The alternative materials (bonded resins and porcelains) are safer and protect the tooth better than amalgam.

You must understand what dentists are taught to understand why they don't think they have to change.

A mercury amalgam filling is not bonded into the tooth cavity. So what prevents decay bacteria from getting between the tooth structure and the filling? We were taught that, immediately after being put into the tooth, a mercury filling begins *to corrode*. It's this corrosion—this rust, in effect—that seals the space between the tooth and the filling with corrosion products. The corrosion debris helps prevent bacteria and saliva from getting under the filling and causing sensitivity in the tooth or causing new decay to form. Let me emphasize that we were taught that uncontrolled debris prevents decay from forming.

In reality, the corrosion of the filling materials causes the amalgam surface to release even more mercury into the mouth. Again, think of a piece of unpainted machinery left out in the rain. You have an alloy in a wet environment—even worse in the mouth where the saliva is often acidic. As seen in Figure 1-20, page 111, the alloy rusts—corrodes—and metals are given off to the surrounding environment. These metals in the mouth are swallowed and inhaled into the body.

But in the case of an amalgam filling, corrosion also causes expansion pressure against the sides of the tooth. Simply biting on the filling for several years will cause compression and movement of the alloy. Think of a blacksmith pounding on a horseshoe to make the metal widen and expand. The bite in your mouth is compressing the amalgam and causing it to expand in a similar manner. But in a rigid tooth, expansion of the filling causes cracking of the enamel and dentin structure around it. This pressure builds up and eventually breaks the tooth or causes the tooth to hurt.

Amalgam fillings in teeth crack and break the tooth until pain or a broken piece call for a dental repair.

Look at Figure 1-21. You can see a small amalgam filling in the top (occlusal) of a first premolar. On both sides of the filling, against the next teeth, you can see black crack lines going down between the teeth.

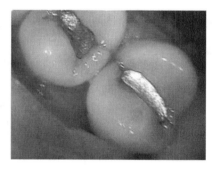

In the second picture, Figure 1-22, after I removed the filling, you can see that the crack line was not just on the top.

Figure 1-21 Expansion of amalgam fractures teeth

The crack extended all the way under the old amalgam filling to the base. This tooth was painful when the person bit down on food. The crack underneath the filling was the cause of the pain, but the *expansion of the mercury filling is what caused the crack to develop*. At any time, the patient could have bitten a hard candy or pretzel and broken off the cracked tooth. The hard food

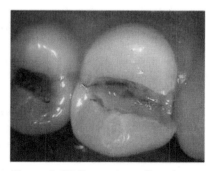

Figure 1-22 Expansion of amalgam fractures teeth

got the blame but the old amalgam set up the fracture.

THE TOXIC DENTAL OFFICE

In a 2005 policy paper on mercury in health care, the World Health Organization (WHO) states that

> dental amalgam is the main source of mercury exposure in non-industrialized settings, exposing the concerned population to mercury level significantly exceeding those set for food and air.

Patients put themselves at risk simply by walking into some dental offices. Exposure to toxic mercury vapor is more probable if the dentist is still placing mercury-amalgam fillings in new cavities. (Remember, estimates are that 50% of dentists are still placing new mercury-amalgam fillings). However even if the dentist does not use this filling material, simply drilling out an old mercury-amalgam without taking safety precautions results in a tremendous increase in the mercury vapor released into the patient's mouth, the surrounding air and the office furnishings themselves. The percentage increase in vapor from the spray and aerosol generated during the drilling out the filling can be 10 to 100 times the resting mercury-vapor levels. The vapor thus released is inhaled and absorbed

◆ by the patient
◆ by the dentist and assistants
◆ into the room surfaces
◆ into the office furnishings
◆ into the office air.

The Toxic Dentist Is Everywhere

In 1985 and 1986, in order to prove they were right—that mercury is not accumulating in dentists who remove (or place) dental amalgam fillings—the American Dental Association conducted a test at one of their annual conventions. Dentists attending the meeting were asked to give a urine sample for a mercury-level test. The overwhelming results of that study showed very few dentists had high levels of mercury in their urine. The ADA proudly announced the study results as proof of the safety and stability of amalgam. Some authors noted a decline of mercury levels in the mid 1980s, which they attributed to less use of mercury amalgam fillings and better handling of the metal.

But we've already seen how mercury is absorbed into the body and how a simple urine test will usually show *no* mercury levels, or minimal levels at most. The mercury is hiding in the body tissues, working on a cellular level to inhibit normal body functions. Dentists and their staffs who are exposed to mercury every day may have mercury toxicity symptoms that they're not aware of. Some studies, including several sponsored by the ADA, have been poorly designed, either not looking at the various sources of mercury that can be absorbed, not looking at all routes of excretion, not accounting for all the confounding factors that might influence test results, not accounting for the environmental factors that might influence test results, or simply not forming accurate conclusions. It is important to remember that most clinicians—either physicians or dentists—do not understand how mercury is metabolized and stored in the body and why there are low circulating levels in body fluids. (See the cardiovascular effects of mercury, below.)

Nonetheless, well designed studies of dentists and health professionals that looked at mercury concentrations in the pituitary and thyroid glands uniformly show a greater exposure to mercury as a result of drilling out old fillings and placing new ones as compared to levels in the general public. Mercury levels are loosely proportional to the number of hours the dentists work per week. The level of mercury in urine and plasma has been found to be proportional to the number of amalgam filling surfaces the dentist places routinely in his office.

In a 1995 study, a DMPS mercury urine challenge test was given to dentists and non-dental personnel. The results are tabulated in the chart below.

**Comparison of Dental Worker vs.
Non-Dental Worker Mercury Levels**

Values are micrograms mercury of urinary excretion

	Before DMPS	After DMPS
Dental Technicians	4.84	424.0
Dentists	3.28	162.0
Non-Dental Personnel	0.78	27.3

These results show dentists and dental personnel to have significant body burdens of mercury as a result of working with the toxic filling material. The circulating mercury in their bodies is 20 times the level of non-dental personnel. This indicates a high probability that *regular dentists' motor and visual capabilities are compromised from mercury toxicity*. Scientific studies have shown serious neurological effects in dentists with an average of 5.5 years in practice, with significantly poorer performance on:

♦ sensory reaction (speed)

♦ motor speed (movement)

♦ visual scanning

♦ visuomotor coordination and concentration

♦ digit (finger) mobility

♦ visual memory (delayed recall)

♦ higher degree of aggressive behavior

♦ higher anxiety levels

♦ confusion and fatigue.

These neurological effects were proportional to length of time in practice and amount of exposure to mercury in the office. A 1982 study of 298 dentists concluded that

> dentists and dental assistants have deficits in motor function
> and cognitive scores in relation to their number of fillings and
> to their urinary mercury excretion…the use of mercury as a
> restorative material is a health risk for dentists.

On the basis of these findings, we are entitled to wonder if such neurological effects might not explain the high incidence of depression and suicide among dentists?

The Toxic Dental Assistant Is Everywhere

Sitting in a dental operatory, assisting a dentist placing (or removing without precautions) mercury amalgams, is hazardous to the dentist's assistant. The California legislature declared in an assembly bill in 2003:

> Infertility and miscarriage levels in dental assistants are both elevated, and all dentists, both male and female, are similarly affected.

Mercury is among the most recognized of the "persistent, bioaccumulative toxicants" —substances that accumulate in the food chain and pose magnified hazards to mammals and humans. Mercury can be a neurotoxin at low doses, affecting the functioning and development of the nervous system. Pregnant women are especially vulnerable to mercury contamination through direct exposure to developing fetuses via the placenta. Children poisoned by mercury show lowered intelligence, impaired hearing and poor coordination according to East Bay Municipal Utility District.

In a 1994 study of 418 female dental assistants, the probability of conception of the assistants was only 63% compared to women not exposed to mercury. The study found two major influences on the severity of the lack of fertility:

1 The more mercury filling exposure per week, the higher the infertility level

2 The more precautions taken to protect the staff from the mercury filling exposure, the lower the infertility level

A 1987 study showed female dentists and dental assistants had more reproductive failures (spontaneous abortions, stillbirths, congenital malformations) and irregular, painful, or hemorrhagic menstrual disorders than a control (unexposed) group of women.

Infertility and miscarriage levels in dental assistants are both elevated, and all dentists, both male and female, are similarly affected.

The dental assistant's exposure to mercury while working on a patient can have the same negative health outcomes as are produced by exposure to mercury by any other means.

And although it's not widely publicized, the simple cleaning of a patient's teeth—as performed in every dental office, exposes the operator to toxic elemental mercury. The process of polishing the surfaces of the teeth abrades and heats up any mercury fillings, thereby elevating the vapor levels in the mouth. As we know, patients with mercury-amalgam fillings have elemental mercury levels in their mouths, while those without amalgam fillings do not. But a study in 1995 in Seattle, Washington (among others) showed that organic and inorganic mercury, usually present in the saliva of a mercury-filling patient before a dental cleaning, is converted to elemental mercury *by the cleaning*. The dental assistant is exposed to this elemental mercury during the cleaning procedure.

The Toxic Dental Office Is Everywhere

Patients entering a dental office have no objective way of judging whether adequate precautions are being taken to maintain a clean environment. We all know that there exist government regulations, guidelines and controls designed to reduce the risk of infectious or hazardous exposures in health-care facilities. We also know that humans make mistakes and patterns of behavior are not easily changed. This laxity of compliance applies to some dental offices too.

The US Occupationl Safety and Health Administration regulations are designed to protect the employees of an office, and these precautions can extend to protection for the patients as well. However in surgical and dental offices, where surgery and exposure to bodily fluids is common, additional precautions must be constantly taken. Basic infection-control protocols must be followed to prevent contamination or infection between all patients and staff. Biological waste must be separately contained in appropriate plastic bags and containers until disposed of properly. Equipment and instruments must be handled with careful procedures as must the treatment of room surfaces. All possible instruments and equipment that can be sterilized must be sterilized.

The mercury released from the filling has to go somewhere. Mercury that isn't swallowed or inhaled by the patient or staff, or isn't sucked away by the assistant suction device, remains in the room. It settles on the room surfaces and walls and gets into the furniture, curtains and flooring. If the office cannot open its windows, as is the case in many new office buildings today, the contaminated air is recirculated

> Dental offices that advertise they do not use mercury amalgam fillings to fill teeeth, but instead use white bonded materials, may still be toxic to patients. If the dentist continues to take out old mercury fillings under less than stringent conditions, the result is a huge increase in mercury vapor through the office.

through the entire office over and over by the heating and air conditioning systems. The mercury off gasses continually from where it has settled, continuously exposing anyone in the office.

The Toxic Dental Patient Is Everywhere

Ask the important questions before you commit as a patient. We've surveyed plenty of studies that have shown that the dentist, assistant and office staff have been exposed to mercury, so you know you will be exposed also. Absorbed mercury in the plasma reduces at a 88-day half-life. In the bladder it is 46 days (with a good excretory system). Half-life means one-half of the original amount will still be present after that time—it will not be totally gone.

There are a number of questions that you must ask your prospective dentist for your own safety.

1. Do you place mercury amalgam fillings in new cavities? (If so, go to a different dentist.)

2. When the old mercury fillings are drilled out what precautions do you take to protect me, the patient, from the toxic vapor?

3. What precautions do you take to protect you (the dentist) and your staff from the vapor? (Will they protect you adequately if they don't protect themselves?)

4. What type of gloves do you use? (Latex gloves allow mercury to pass through into the skin; gloves must be nitrile or synthetic.)

5. Do you alter your treatment recommendations depending upon my sensitivities and the overall health of each patient or does everyone get their fillings replaced the same way?

6. Do you clean the office air of residual toxic and noxious odors and VOCs (volatile organic compounds) that can cause me to get sick? How do you do that? (This is especially important if the office cannot open their windows.)

7. Do you have an amalgam separator in your waste line to capture mercury runoff and protect the drinking water and environment? (If they don't care about protecting the water supply, do they care about your overall health?)

OUT WITH THE OLD

Curtis had not been to a dentist for three years. He finally decided to take the plunge because some of his teeth had chipped. He was a smart 46-year-old but, like so many of my new patients, he had tried to put off seeing a dentist because it wasn't fun. There's the expense. There's the time involved.

There's the fear of pain during the visit.

This last one was Curtis' reason. I talked with him for over 30 minutes about his health needs. We discussed his past medical and dental histories and talked about what he wanted me to do for him and his dental health. I advised him about basic nutrition and vitamin and mineral supplements he might consider taking to help his overall health. He was basically healthy with no symptoms of any significance. He had no allergies and was taking no medication.

I examined his mouth and teeth and then performed an oral mercury vapor test with our atomic spectrometer. I sat down on my dental stool.

"Curtis, you have eight teeth with mercury amalgam fillings in them. You have a total of fourteen surfaces of mercury fillings all together." I explained how the mercury off-gasses from the fillings constantly and how his body absorbs and excretes the toxic metal.

"Just sitting there, you have an oral mercury-vapor level of 9.6 micrograms per cubic meter. When you chew or drink hot or acidic beverages or anything you might do to activate the filling surfaces, your vapor level goes up to 41.0. This is...it's a high level in a person's mouth, Curtis. The inhalation limit imposed by the EPA for inhaled mercury is only 9.0 micrograms per cubic meter. Plus most of these fillings have cracks and decay and need to be restored."

Over the following two years Curtis had all the necessary dental restorations completed. He finished in June and I saw him again in October during his routine 6-month dental checkup. I examined his mouth and after not finding any problem, I was about to leave the room when he stopped me.

"Dr. Robbins, the strangest thing happened since I saw you last June. I never mentioned it to you at that time but for over 15 years. I've had pain in my feet and ankles when I bend them, like when I stretch before exercising. Over the last few years the pain had progressed to my knees. It was so painful I consulted with several doctors including a rheumatologist. They performed every test they could think of but could find no reason for the pain." He stood and demonstrated the normal flexing and extending of his knees that was painful. It was not an extreme bending by any means. "The funny thing was, I could do exercise like running without pain. It was only when I bent my ankles or knees slightly more that the pain began.

"Anyway, I noticed the last few weeks that the pain is gone. I didn't realize it at first, then I thought it would come back. But it didn't. I'm sure it's related to the mercury that was in my mouth. Once you removed the last two mercury fillings four months ago, the pain left. I can hardly believe it!"

Is it worth having your mercury-amalgam fillings removed and replaced? Unequivocally, yes. Will it improve your health? Will it make you feel better? My personal opinion is yes although I cannot guarantee the specific result. You *must* remove all mercury (and other metals we'll look at later) from your mouth as soon as possible. Why?

♦ Removing the toxic mercury fillings and crowns from your mouth will prevent additional mercury accumulation in your body tissues and fluids.

♦ Measured mercury in all body fluids is reduced after the fillings are removed. Decreased mercury levels are noted in the blood, plasma and urine.

♦ Removal will stop your long-term chronic exposure to mercury, exposure that can lead to impairment of brain function and disease.

♦ Scientific and medical studies have demonstrated that, when the dental fillings are removed, ill health due to mercury exposure is reduced.

♦ Patients report to doctors *an improved quality of life* after the removal of amalgam fillings.

♦ Damage to your tooth structure from the expanding amalgam fillings will stop.

♦ Damage to your tooth structure under full crowns, whether gold with metals or covered with porcelain, will stop. The crowns' direct contact with mercury fillings underneath causes damage to the tooth and the release of more mercury (galvanic current as described earlier). *Removing the damaging mercury fillings will help preserve the remaining tooth structure.*

♦ Bonding white restorations in place of the old mercury amalgams will strengthen the teeth.

BUT SAFELY!

Your immediate objective should be to lessen your chances of mercury exposure and toxicity. An important part of that is your choice of a dentist who adheres to basic safe amalgam-removal protocols. Some of the protocols I use in my own practice, called Bio-SafeDentistry, are part of the standard of care for the International Academy of Oral Medicine and Toxicology (www.iaomt.org), This is an organization whose members are guided by scientific and medical evidence in the practice of modern safe dentistry.

> Removal [of toxic mercury fillings and crowns] will stop your long-term chronic exposure to mercury, exposure that can lead to impairment of brain function and disease.

HERE ARE MY BASIC BIOSAFEDENTISTRY® PROTOCOLS:

1. Antioxidant and Detoxifier Administration

No matter how many safeguards or devices we use, some mercury released during drilling out of a filling will be absorbed into the patient's body. It may be absorbed through the mucosa of the mouth (just as your skin can absorb elemental mercury) or swallowed with your saliva. Some of the vapor released will be inhaled through the mouth and absorbed through the lungs, even if the patient is breathing inhaled air under positive pressure. My approach is to prepare the body to capture this mercury in the bloodstream before it enters any cellular tissues. Assuming my patient has no serious health problems, I recommend certain supplements, though I always instruct patients to check with their physician about taking the supplements should there be a question or interaction with any medication they are taking. (See supplements at www.biosafedentistry.com) If the patient has only one or two very small mercury amalgam fillings to be removed, I will administer a transdermal reduced glutathione (200 mg) at the time of the removal. I dispense additional doses to the patient with instructions on taking those throughout that day. The glutathione is absorbed through the skin in under one hour and is an effective antioxidant with sulfhydryl groups that latch onto any free mercury in the bloodstream. High doses of vitamin C are essential to help the body excrete the captured mercury before it has a chance to detach from the glutathione and enter the body's fats and liver.

If the patient has a significant number of mercury-amalgam fillings to be removed, and several visits are needed to complete their removal, I recommend a combination of supplements. Reduced glutathione (100-200 mg) is taken orally beginning the day before the appointment and ending the day after. Two doses are taken at a time, twice daily for the total of three days. Alpha lipoic acid (100–200 mg) is taken orally at the same time, with the same number of doses as the reduced glutathione. Alpha lipoic acid is a potent antioxidant that also removes toxins from the body in much the way that glutathione does. To complete the mercury removal from the body, I also recommend high daily doses of vitamin C (L-ascorbic acid)—3 to 8 gm each day. Vitamin C, a potent antioxidant and free radical scavenger, assists in the excretion of the mercury via the patient's urine and stool. Because ascorbic acid can induce acid indigestion, I recommend a buffered C powder. This virtually eliminates any acid indigestion effect. I will occasionally recommend selenium also.

I will sometimes recommend zeolite, a product that is chemically inert, yet is said to capture toxins and heavy metals in the body. Once captured, the toxic molecules are excreted in the stool. This can be used as an adjunct for removal of mercury absorbed by the body. (See Natural Cellular Defense at www.mywaiora.com/771401)

Some dentists will use chlorella, a natural chelating agent derived from algae. (www.vitacost.com) Homeopathic remedies are especially useful, depending upon the patient's toxicity.

How to Take Vitamin C. The human body cannot produce vitamin C so you must ingest it each day in your diet. It is rapidly utilized once ingested, and within hours, any ascorbic acid not used is excreted. If too much is taken at one time, stomach gurgles will result and diarrhea may follow. It is therefore necessary to take the three to 8 gm of vitamin C each day *in divided doses*. Each person's body metabolism and toxic level is different. Not only will each person require a different amount of Vitamin C each day, but their own amounts taken will vary from day to day as well. The vitamin C is started five days before the removal appointment so the patient can adjust their dose for comfort. It is continued for five days following the removal, although I recommend they stay on the vitamin, for overall health, indefinitely.

2. Removal Method

Dentists should try to remove old fillings in several large pieces. This exposes patients to less mercury vapor than drilling the entire filling out in tiny particles, causing more aerosol and vaporization to inhale and swallow.

3. High Speed Suction

The dental assistant should keep the large suction tube in the mouth throughout the entire procedure. Large amounts of water must be used to keep flushing out the debris and aerosols. The vapor and aerosols suctioned out of the mouth should be vented to the outside of the building, while the particles, debris and amalgam sludge should be captured by the mercury separator in the building.

4. Rubber Dam

There is some question as to whether a rubber dam should be used or not. A rubber dam is used by some dentists to isolate the tooth being worked on. A hole is made in the sheet of latex (or vinyl) and placed over the tooth. All procedures performed on the tooth are effectively on one side of the dam, while the patient is on the other side with a saliva ejector in their mouth, sucking up fluids from around the tongue. In my opinion, with the latex sheet covering the mouth, it is not possible for the dental assistant to effectively suction out the mercury and vapor in the mouth, so the patient inhales, absorbs or swallows it. It has also been shown that mercury can penetrate the latex dam and end up in the mouth anyway.

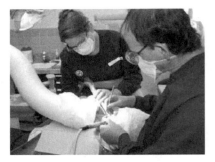

Figure 1-23: Patient has the skin on their face and head covered with damp drapes to prevent mercury contact and absorption.

5. Cover the Skin

Mercury can pass right through the skin. That is why mercury thermometers can be so dangerous. They can break and children (and some adults too!) play with the liquid mercury or just get it on their skin. It gets absorbed through the skin and right into the body tissues and bloodstream.

When removing mercury-amalgam fillings we drape the exposed areas of the patients face and head with damp towels to avoid exposure from mercury spray landing on the skin.

6. Sterile Gloves

Mercury can pass through latex and vinyl gloves, so the doctor must wear synthetic gloves (nitrile) to avoid exposure.

7. Breathing Air

There is no completely effective way for the patient to avoid breathing in some of the contaminated air while the filling is removed. That's why I use the antioxidant supplements. To help reduce inhalation of these vapors, however, I may fit the patient with a nose hood that allows them to breathe central air or oxygen from a compressed gas tank. The supplemental air can be administered with a positive air pressure to help displace air exhausted from the drilling that would otherwise be inhaled by the patient.

8. Respirators for the Staff

The air space surrounding the patient's mouth is contaminated with mercury aerosols and vapor while drilling. To reduce the inhalation of this vapor, some dentists (and staff) will wear a respirator mask that has cartridges through which air breathed in is filtered. Special cartridges must be used to capture the mercury vapor specifically. They are cumbersome and not easy to use, but they do protect the staff against mercury exposure.

An alternate method is the use of a positive pressure respirator. This is a smaller mask worn by the staff and connected to a compressed gas tank of air. This air can be the same air tank from which the patient is breathing.

From my research I have found that using the IQAir Dental Hg FlexVac mercury air cleaner, the one shown in action below, eliminates all ambient mercury vapor released around the patient's mouth during the procedure. My atomic spectrometer shows no measurable levels of vapor within one foot of the filling being removed. We consequently do not use respirators for the staff.

9. Air in the Treatment Room

As we've seen, mercury vapor and particles are aerated and sprayed from the mouth during the drilling of the tooth. This aerosol contains toxic mercury and can be inhaled by anyone in the room. The use of a mercury filtration device is essential to avoid the gross exposure. Figure 1-24 shows the best unit available, in my opinion, after much research. The IQAir Dental Mercury FlexVac is a Swiss-made, medical-grade high efficiency mercury air cleaner. (See www.biologicaircleaners.com) It pulls in aerosols at over 260 cubic feet per minute and helps keep the entire room free of mercury aerosols. I was so impressed by its solid design and the university studies proving its effectiveness at capturing mercury vapor that I became a dealer for their use in dental offices. Very few dentists were using this type of filtration unit when I started promoting its use. (SMARTAir Solutions 888-9779-AIR)

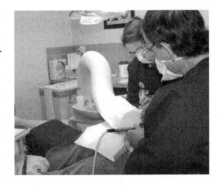

Figure 1-24: This IQAir Mercury FlexVac unit captures 99.8% of the mercury vapor passing through the tube.

The mercury air cleaner also absorbs much of the volatile organic compounds and off-gassing coming from any of the other chemicals we use in the operatory. That includes many of the disinfection and sterilization chemicals that are essential for infection control, but may not be healthy to inhale. If a unit such as this is keeping the room air clean, it is also helping keep the dental staff and the patient from exposure.

In my opinion, dentists using a negative ion generator or an electrostatic precipitator are not doing an effective or safe job. In order to capture some of the contaminants, these units must pull the contaminated vapor across the room, across the staff's faces and across your nose. That is far too much opportunity for exposure. Worse, the electrostatic plates lose considerable effectiveness soon after going into operation, since a thin film of contaminants land on the electrode surfaces and prevent further capture. Cleaning these plates is a dirty and toxic job.

10. Air in the Whole Office

The dental office as a whole can be sick, contaminated with mercury or other toxic compounds that can cause bad reactions in anyone coming into the office. The ambient office air may also contain pollen and allergens that can trigger allergic reactions, as well as bacteria and viruses.

IQAir makes another high efficiency air cleaner, the IQAir DentalPro, which sits in the office corridor or a large room and filters the air 24 hours, day and night. This assures that any toxic vapor or particles escaping from the treatment rooms are captured and held to prevent patients having a bad physical reaction to them. The office will be free of bad odors.

The United States Department of Health and Human Services, in its 2005 Priority Substance List of the most hazardous substances, ranks mercury as third after arsenic and lead.

MERCURY AFFECTS THE WHOLE BODY

The symptoms of mercury exposure and toxicity are, of course, related to which system is affected in the body. But there are universal symptoms, especially with long-term exposure.

Some of the toxic effects of mercury have been discussed and illustrated in the actual patient cases I've included throughout this book. Governmental agencies set what are claimed as "acceptable limits of mercury exposure based upon *clinical evidence*." In other words if someone is sick from an exposure of 50 micrograms of inhaled mercury vapor, then 50 micrograms goes into the statistic pool as too high an amount. But as we've already seen, there has never been a safe level of mercury exposure established and a World Health Organization scientific panel as early as 1991 concluded the only safe level of mercury in the body below which no adverse effects could be found is zero.

Once mercury is absorbed into the blood stream it is within minutes converted into an organic form, methylmercury. Methylmercury is rapidly absorbed into fatty tissues and the liver and kidneys. It is further dispersed into all other body cells, including the cell nucleus and mitochondria, where it disrupts enzyme and energy production. It causes specific effects in the body depending upon which enzymes are affected.

In 2003 the US Centers for Disease Control and Prevention reported one in 12 (8%) of American women of childbearing age had mercury in their blood above the levels considered safe by the EPA. This is 4.7 *million women* and puts *322,000 newborns at risk for neurological deficits each year*. This estimate has recently been recalculated to be almost twice this number.

> Pregnant women and nursing mothers with mercury amalgam dental fillings must not have any non-emergency dental work performed.

Pregnant women and nursing mothers cannot risk exposure to methylmercury. Studies have shown this organic mercury accumulates in the baby and breast milk and affects the levels of noradrenalin and nerve growth factor in the developing brains of offspring. Inorganic mercury exposure from dental amalgams causes increased mercury in blood and breast milk. And, by the way, exposure to methylmercury from eating fish was *not* reflected in breast milk!

What can *low* levels of mercury vapor do to a developing fetus? A 1995 study showed *low level mercury vapor can change the level of nerve growth factors and its receptors in the brain of fetuses*. It can cause neuronal (nerve) damage and disturbed trophic (growth) regulations during development.

Mercury accumulates in the body tissues and is difficult to remove. Consequently long-time buildup will cause more advanced health effects, which will become permanent. The earlier that absorbed mercury is removed from the body, the sooner further toxic exposure and injuries from the exposure will cease. Some observed health effects may still be present while others may heal or reverse towards normal function.

It's for all these reasons that many states and cities have enacted informed-consent requirements for dentists to assure that dentists tell their patients that mercury is going into their teeth—and their bodies.

◖◗

Freya Koss is now a 65-year-old politically active woman, sharp as a tack. She was not always like this.

In 1998, during a routine dental examination, she was told she had a cavity. She needed a filling so the dentist drilled out the old amalgam filling and placed a new mercury-amalgam filling in the tooth. Later that week while attending a ballet performance, she became dizzy and experienced double vision while driving home. Not knowing what was wrong she consulted several physicians and had many tests performed. She received diagnoses of everything from lupus erythematosis (an autoimmune disease where the body attacks its own tissues), to multiple sclerosis. When her right eyelid began to droop, they diagnosed her with myasthenia gravis. She was told she would never be normal again.

She began searching the internet and discovered many other people with similar health problems. All these people had one thing in common. They all had dental work, specifically mercury amalgam fillings, performed before their health went downhill. There were hundreds of websites from physicians, dentists, scientists and the general public relating the connections between all sorts of medical diagnoses with dental mercury amalgams. All their cases were misdiagnosed by doctors who did not understand heavy metal toxicity and its effects on the human body, especially mercury poisoning from dental fillings.

She sought out one of the few biologic dentists who knew how to carefully and safely remove old mercury-amalgam fillings and replace them with bonded white ones. It took months of dental treatment. After they were replaced, she needed to detoxify her body, so she was treated by an integrative physician who knew about mercury poisoning. After *four years of treatment* Freya felt better than she had for many years. Her "brain fog" was gone and she reported a surge in energy, though she still reports occasional double vision and some ocular muscle weakness.

Freya has become an anti-mercury activist. She was put off by her past physicians and dentists who ignored the evidence in the scientific literature and her case study in particular. Freya has organized many groups and professionals to politically change dental care in the United States. She is saddened that the American Dental Association has been lying to their members and the public about the dangers of mercury amalgam dental fillings for years.

"I'm sorry for dentists," she says. "They think they're helping people when, in fact, they're harming them, their office workers and themselves."

She's angry that the state dental boards, which are populated by members of the American Dental Association, have tried for years to pull the licenses of dentists who tell their patients the truth about mercury in dental fillings and the health consequences of using them.

Freya Koss is now the development director for Consumers for Dental Choice, Wynnewood, PA and the PA Coalition for Mercury-Free Dentistry. She can be reached at www.toxicteeth.org.

ﻌﻌ

Mercury Poisoning: Why Some and Not Others?

The American Dental Association has made a point of taking two people with the same number of mercury amalgam fillings and saying, "Look at these two people. They have the same number of fillings yet one is sick and one is healthy. It clearly cannot be the mercury in their fillings that is the cause of all the health problems."

But the truth is that the efficiency with which a person's body can excrete toxins, including mercury, and get them out of their body will determine if that person exhibits health problems and dysfunction. A person with a good enzyme and catalyst system will avoid much of the immediate damage to their body systems. *It is to a great extent a matter of genetics whether you have good excretion or not.* Echeverria and associates recently reported that polymorphisms of the gene encoding urinary porphyrin excretion (coproporphyrinogen oxidase [CPOX4]), altered the impact of mercury on cognitive and mood scores. Approximately 25% of the US population is polymorphic for this genotype. In other words variations in a gene will determine the extent of damage to the psychological framework and awareness of the individual.

In the ADA's straw-man example, the sick person with mercury amalgam fillings cannot in fact excrete mercury fast enough to avoid a body buildup and subsequent disease. However, if there is an overwhelming exposure to mercury, no amount of genetic coding can get the mercury out fast enough and you will show toxic symptoms sooner or later.

How Mercury Affects the Body's Various Systems

The Cardiovascular System

Acute exposure to mercury can cause tachycardia (fast heart rate) and hypertension (high blood pressure). Inhalation exposure to mercury vapor causes increased blood pressure and heart palpitations.

A 1955 study of Finnish men showed that accumulation of mercury in the body is associated with an excess risk of a heart attack (acute myocardial infarction). Other studies show high mercury levels in cardiac muscle tissue with increased incidence of arrhythmias and cardiomyopathies (heart muscle dysfunction). The concentration of mercury in the cardiac muscle itself in patients with cardiomyopathies was 22,000 times greater than those without the heart pathology.

> A study in Finnish men showed an increased risk of heart attack, arrhythmias, and cardiomyopathies—and a 22,000-fold higher concentration of mercury in the heart muscle of patients with cardiomyopathies compared to those without cardiomyopathy.

Results of another study, in 2003 at a University in Brazil, indicate "that cardiac effects may be observed after continuous exposure to very small concentrations of mercury, probably as a result of the [myocardial muscle] cell capacity to concentrate mercury. These results also indicate that continuous professional exposure to mercury followed by its absorption might have toxicological consequences affecting cardiac function, and being considered hazardous."

The Gastrointestinal System

Acute exposure—including exposure in the mouth to inhalation of mercury vapor—can lead to excessive salivation, difficulty swallowing and burning of the lining of the mouth. Abdominal pain, nausea and diarrhea are also possible consequences. But damage to the gastrointestinal tract can extend to leaky gut syndrome, the inability to absorb nutrients properly that befell Janet, whose story I told at the start of this chapter. It can lead to more serious conditions such as Crohn's disease, ulcerative colitis and inflammatory bowel disease (IBS).

The Immune System

Cheryl, a 39-year-old married mother of three, located our office on the Internet and drove four hours to see me. She was appointed for a new patient examination and waited in my treatment room.

After introductions were made, I asked her what concerns she had come to see me about. She was obviously tired but glad that she was finally doing something about her health. She hadn't seen a dentist for over five years.

"I've had a bad few years," she began. "I have had chronic fatigue syndrome, mental fog and severe pre-menstrual syndrome. I'm depressed. I clean houses for a living and can barely make it through the day I'm so tired.

"My physician ordered a urine challenge test a few months ago and it came back with high levels of mercury, copper and some other metals. He started to do some IV [intravenous] chelation to get the mercury out but I didn't react real well. I figured why get the mercury out of my body if there are tons of it in my teeth? Dr. Robbins, shouldn't I get the mercury fillings replaced before I do any chelation?"

I really like it when my patients are well-informed and have done their homework. It makes the consultation more effective because they already know what I am talking about.

"You're absolutely right Cheryl. Why remove mercury from the body when the teeth will put it right back into your tissues?"

She nodded in agreement. "I stopped the treatments and consulted with someone in my area who treats patients nutritionally and understands toxic metal disease. She's a nutritional doctor and after seeing me she placed me on several supplements to help my body cope with my stresses and problems. She recommended I get a biologic dentist to safely remove the mercury dental fillings as soon as possible. She thought that alone might make me feel better. But I couldn't find a dentist anywhere near me who was concerned about putting mercury in patients' teeth."

After examining her mouth I took an oral mercury vapor reading. It showed a minimal resting mercury level because she had not had her teeth polished for so long that they were slightly covered with plaque and calculus. However when she chewed for three minutes and was tested again, her level went up to 10.1, a moderately high level. During the consultation Cheryl was told it would cost over $6,000 to replace her mercury fillings with bonded restorations. She expected as much.

"I knew it was going to be expensive since I didn't have any dental work for years. I have to do this for myself because I cannot function anymore the way I feel. My kids need braces but they will have to wait. If I can't work nobody will get anything!"

I respected Cheryl's decision to improve her health. I also understood how important this was to her because she not only was travelling hours each way, but also she was postponing her children's dental care. Over the next seven months we removed all the mercury from her mouth and replaced the fillings.

Several months after the procedures were completed, Cheryl came in for a routine dental checkup. I noticed she seemed different and told her she looked much better than the last time she was in the office. She smiled.

"Dr. Robbins, I feel really good. Getting that mercury out really made a difference. I'm so much more energetic and I don't get as tired as I was. I never could have gotten through this last year the way I was. I want to thank you for helping me clear this up!"

I smiled and told her that committing to all the dental work was to her credit. It was the means to her improving her health.

☙

The body normally prevents pathogens from passing through the gut wall. But with an intestinal system that is compromised by the effects of mercury, these pathogens can now enter the body. Body cells that are now less resistant are open to attack, thus overworking the immune system. This chronic exposure and fighting of inflammation and pathogens can be debilitating to the body, leading to chronic fatigue and other inflammatory conditions.

There is evidence suggesting autoimmune diseases may be caused by mercury exposure, and other evidence suggesting that patients with many amalgam fillings have more antibiotic-resistant bacteria. These patients have a harder time fighting all kinds of infections in their bodies, because traditional antibiotics will not work against these bugs.

Some good news. One study, conducted in 2004 at the Institute of Dental Research, of the Czech Republic, examined patients with certain autoimmune and allergic diseases such as systemic lupus, multiple sclerosis, autoimmune thyroiditis or atopic eczema. Six months after replacement of their mercury amalgam fillings, 71% of the subjects exhibited improved health. This is consistent with other studies showing removal of mercury amalgam fillings lowers mercury exposure in the body.

The Neurological System

The central nervous system and brain are most at risk for permanent injury from mercury-vapor exposure. Although methylmercury crosses the blood-brain barrier, once in the brain it is converted to inorganic mercury. This form is the most difficult to remove. If mercury infiltrates the brain, it causes destruction of the tubulin protective covering of nerve axons, which leads to nerve-cell death (as in the case of Alzheimer's disease and some fatigue syndromes). Consequently it has been suggested as a primary risk factor for multiple sclerosis

> A Swedish study showed psychiatric disorders in 87% of individuals with mercury-amalgam dental fillings and 6% of individuals without dental work.

and Alzheimer's disease. An association has been demonstrated between a body burden of mercury and Parkinson's disease. Other nerve and muscle dysfunction can also appear as tremors, rashes or muscle weakness.

Because much of the permanent and serious neurological damage is due to long-term *chronic* exposure to mercury, the effects of mercury vapor from dental fillings has been clouded by other sources of exposure that are more obvious.

Early *acute* neurological symptoms include: (see Appendix A for symptoms of exposure)

♦ Tremors, starting in the hands but gradually affecting other parts of the body.

♦ Emotional lability: This symptom is common in cases of brain injury and includes uncontrollable actions that may be inappropriate or cause embarrassment and social avoidance. Examples are irritability, shyness, confidence loss, crying or laughter and nervousness.

♦ Insomnia

♦ Memory loss

♦ Weakness, muscle atrophy (wasting), twitching

♦ Headaches

♦ Abnormal sensations in hands with abnormal reflexes elsewhere

♦ Deficient performances in everyday actions (cognitive functions).

Chronic exposure to mercury can lead to

♦ Unsteady walking

♦ Poor concentration

♦ Shaky speech

♦ Blurred vision

♦ Poor motor skills

♦ Slowed nerve responses

♦ Behavioral changes.

In a 1977 Swedish study of 131 subjects, patients' performance related to mercury release during dental restorations, showed psychiatric disorders in 87% as opposed to 6% of those not having dental work. The anxiety, muscular tension, behavioral actions and neuroses including phobias (fears) and obsessions could not be explained by any medical finding.

Many clinicians have noted a possible connection between mercury exposure from dental fillings and multiple sclerosis (MS). One study in 1997 showed significant blood changes in MS subjects with amalgam fillings as compared to MS subjects without amalgam fillings. The MS mercury fillings group had lower levels of red blood cells, hemoglobin and hematocrit. Their thyroxine (T_4) levels were lower, as were their total T-lymphocytes and T-8 (CD8) suppressor cells. The mercury amalgam group also had higher blood urea nitrogen (BUN) and BUN/creatinine ratios, with lower serum immunoglobulin G. *These are major changes signifying a direct connection between mercury amalgam dental fillings and multiple sclerosis.*

Ophthalmic System

High levels of mercury as exhibited by high urinary mercury excretion has been shown to induce a color-vision loss. Expressed as a color confusion index (CCI) urinary excretion in the 50+ micro-grams per gram creatinine level indicates the presence of high levels of mercury which causes vision loss in the blue-yellow range.

Another study in 1998 related visual contrast sensitivity to low mercury urinary levels.

Chronic mercury exposure can cause discoloration of the cornea and lens, eyelid tremor and, rarely, disturbances of vision and extraocular muscles.

Renal System

Exposure to mercury predictably causes dysfunction in the kidneys since mercury is cleared in part through the kidneys. Tissue necrosis (i.e., tissue death) can occur with renal failure.

Elemental mercury vapor has caused spilling of protein in the urine, decreased urine production and blood in the urine.

A 1989 report of the autopsy of three dentists revealed a three times higher amount of mercury in the kidneys than in unexposed subjects.

Reproductive System

Elemental mercury has the ability to cross the placental barrier and infants may also be exposed to mercury from a nursing mother's milk.

Respiratory System

Acute exposure leads within a few hours to difficulty breathing, chest pain and a dry cough. Flu-like symptom can develop and, if severe, can progress to pulmonary edema, respiratory failure and death. If the episode subsides and the tissue damage is not severe, the lung damage can resolve completely, although the mercury toxicity in the tissues remains.

PROTECTING YOURSELF IN THE DENTIST OFFICE

There are several ways you can protect yourself from the effects of mercury exposure.

1. Use a dentist who follows the protocols that can keep your mercury exposure minimal during the drilling out of old amalgam fillings and the removal of crowns, both those crowns with toxic metal or ones covering mercury fillings.

2. Look for dental offices using medical-grade high-efficiency mercury air cleaners (IQAir Dental Hg and FlexVac units are among the best) that are running continuously day and night to constantly filter the office air. These cleaners remove not just incidental ambient mercury vapor that might be in the air, but also volatile organic compounds (VOCs), organic and inorganic chemicals from disinfection and sterilization procedures in the office, other odors, bacteria, viruses, and allergens such as pollen and ragweed.

> You must have your mercury fillings removed safely and replaced with bonded restorations. Objective studies (as I note in the above sections) conclusively show improvement in overall health and quality of life after mercury fillings are removed. Many health problems, both serious and moderate, can be resolved and many patients can be restored to good health by the removal of mercury from their bodies.

3. Offices that have amalgam separators on their waste lines are serious about preventing contamination from mercury leaving their offices. If they are serious about the environment, they are probably serious about your overall health.

4. Choose a dental office that has had special continuing education training on biologic dentistry. Running a safe, non-toxic dental

office is *not* taught in dental schools. It requires additional knowledge to recognize the hazards in the office and know how to correct them. I have helped conventional dental offices transition into BioSafe dental practices.

5. The dentist must evaluate each patient individually to determine how extensive the amalgam removal is going to be and how debilitated or ill the patient is at that time, or may be after the removal appointment. Prior to treatment, he or she must discuss with you if there is a need for additional protection from the mercury. Some patients who have a high body burden of mercury or are sick from its effects will need additional help like breathing oxygen during the appointment. Some patients will need to go to a physician immediately after the dental appointment is finished. They might need an intravenous chelation or supportive treatment to keep them from getting sicker while the mercury in their mouths is removed.

6. If you are a pregnant woman or nursing mother, do not have mercury-amalgam fillings or crowns removed unless it is an emergency. Removing the mercury will expose you and the baby excessively and is not worth the risk. Wait until after the birth or after you are finished nursing to have the amalgams in your mouth removed. The US Agency for Toxic Substances and Disease Registry recommends pregnant women NOT have their mercury amalgam fillings removed while pregnant. They state that "the removal of the mercury-amalgam fillings would actually expose the patient to a greater amount of mercury for a while." The baby accumulates mercury at a rate 10 times that of the mother, and it attacks the developing brain and neurological systems. The US Department of Health and Human Services, as early as 1993, recommended minimizing exposure to mercury fillings for

> ...pregnant women and nursing women (to minimize the
> exposure to their developing young), young children up to the

age of six (and especially up to the age of three), people with impaired kidney function, and people with hypersensitive immune response to mercury.

7. Try to be as healthy and active as you can before the removal of your fillings. A patient in good health can resist the effects of mercury exposure far better than onr who has health problems.

8. As directed by a BioSafe dentist or biologic dentist beforehand, take special supplements and vitamins for a few days before the dental appointment. These help capture any incidental mercury absorbed or inhaled during the appointment. Continue the supplements for a few days following the removal of the amalgams.

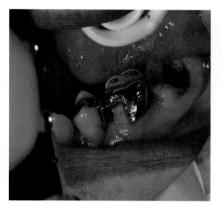

Figure 1-5: Mercury filling under gold alloy causes galvanic shock and increased corrosion. This is not good dentistry.

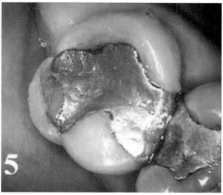

Figure 1-10: Old mercury amalgam in a 2-surface filling damages the tooth and gives off mercury.

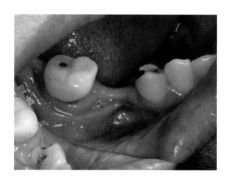

Figure 1-18: Amalgam tattoo from a large mercury filling remaining after tooth extracted.

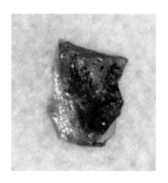

Figure 1-20: Old corroded amalgam removed from tooth

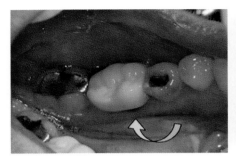

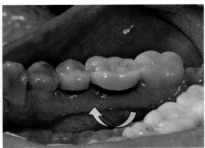

Figure 2-5: The gingiva (gum) has receded away from the metal margin of the crown. This is not seen with the gum on the two adjacent teeth.

Image 2-6: Red and inflamed gingiva around the two metal margins of these crowns only; not present on the other natural teeth

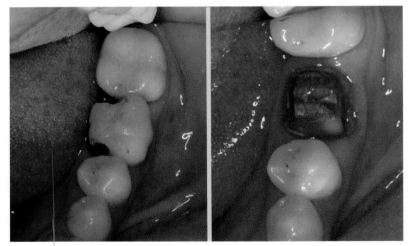

Figure 2-7: Fractured porcelain and metal crown hides toxic mercury amalgam.

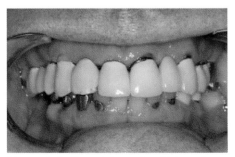

Figure 2-8: Porcelain and gold/metal crowns with exposed margins

2
OTHER METALS

"Metal ions are released from dental alloys into the oral
environment, which can cause biological responses over
short and extended periods."

~ Dr. Liza A. Pon, Associate Professor,
  Dr. Hyeong-Cheol Yang,
   Pon Laboratory,
  Department of Anatomy and Cell Biology,
  Columbia University

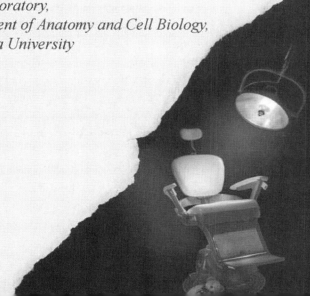

Mark, a 42-year-old accountant from New Brunswick, NJ, came to me for consultation as a last resort. He had been through years of doctors and tests for symptoms that had not improved and had affected his work and his home life. His bouts of depression, mood swings—especially anxiety—frequent headaches, joint pain and fatigue were wearing him down.

He had cardiovascular and rheumatological workups, checks for inflammatory markers, radiological examinations, some tests performed more than once, and various blood tests including tests for Lyme disease and autoimmune diseases. He sat in my examination chair, looking exhausted.

"Two years ago I had all my mercury dental fillings replaced with bonded ones. There were only three fillings but I thought it was worth a try. The dentist took precautions so I wouldn't get worse from their removal. I thought that might help my symptoms but it didn't work.

"After reading the information on your website I thought I would talk to you about my teeth. I was overdue for a checkup anyway so this is a good opportunity to get your take on any oral problems I might still have."

I sat Mark back in the chair and adjusted the dental light. When he opened his mouth, I got a big surprise.

"You have a lot of gold onlays and crowns in your mouth," I said. "It's unusual nowadays to see all this gold in somebody's teeth. People usually want white tooth-colored fillings put in their teeth instead. Where did you have them done?"

"All those gold crowns were placed by a dentist in California over 14 years ago," he explained. "I used to live there until I moved to Pennsylvania."

At the conclusion of my examination, I sat Mark up and considered his case.

"You don't have any visible decay in your mouth or on your x-rays. But the gold restorations block the x-rays, so there may be decay I can't see under any of those. I'm not recommending taking any of them out for that reason. But Mark, the gold in those restorations may not be 100% gold. Pure gold is too soft for most dental uses. It must be alloyed with other metals to strengthen it so it can withstand the pressures of chewing. And these other metals in the gold crowns are like the mercury in your old dental fillings: they can leech out and be absorbed by your body. Some of these can accumulate in your body tissues and some of them are toxic. I'm not saying this is definitely what's going on here but it *can* be a factor in your overall health."

Some patients almost fall asleep when I go into detail about their health. Their eyes almost glaze over. But Mark was interested in what I was saying.

"If you want to check this out, I could remove one of your gold onlays and replace it with a bonded porcelain one. I'd send the old gold to a lab for analysis so we could see what's in the metal."

Mark agreed to the procedure. When I removed a gold onlay the next week, I found decay underneath this one tooth. In two weeks, when he returned for the bonding of the new porcelain onlay, I had the analysis back from the lab. "Look, Mark. The lab result is amazing. This gold alloy contains over 30% copper. That's a tremendous amount considering you have 11 gold restorations in your mouth. Your body is being exposed to high levels of copper and that could be contributing to your symptoms. I can't guarantee that getting all the gold–copper alloy out of your mouth will make you healthy again, but I *can* guarantee that when it's out, you'll not be exposed to the copper anymore."

He agreed to the procedures and a month later there was no more metal in his mouth.

Six months passed before I saw Mark again. He was smiling with renewed energy when he came in for his routine dental checkup. His headaches and joint pain had all but disappeared and he reported he had tons more energy. The physician he was seeing was managing his withdrawal from copper toxicity quite well. He said his wife had commented that he no longer suffered from mood swings and he was generally happier.

ᔆ

When I stopped using mercury in dental fillings in 1982, it never occurred to me that other metals in dentistry might also be sources of toxicity. Even now almost all dentists consider dental–metal alloys safe and inert for use in teeth. But in 1999 I began thinking about this issue.

When a tooth is missing over half its structure due to decay or fracture, restoring it with a bonded filling is not the best treatment choice. White bonded resin fillings are slightly more elastic than tooth structure. If they are used in situations where they are more than half the top of the tooth, the filling will expand and contract at a different rate than the tooth structure, causing micro-cracks and excessive wearing of the filling. This may cause pain when the patient bites down on it. The resin will usually not last as long as a bonded filling should. How long is that? With good oral hygiene and regular dental polishings, a *well-placed bonded resin filling should last well over 10 years.*

When faced with a tooth that is missing 50% or so, most dentists (I would guess over 95%) will recommend that the tooth needs a full crown. Without going into the exact procedure, suffice it to say that after the old filling and decay are removed, the remaining tooth is partially filled and then the entire top is drilled down around all sides and just under the gum, to make room for the crown to cover what is left. Almost all dentists will then recommend a crown made from metal with a porcelain covering fused to it. Dental laboratories use all sorts of metal for this crown. They carry such labels as gold, high noble, low noble, semi-precious, non-precious, etc. When I used to make these types of crowns for patients, I'd always ask the lab for a "gold fused to porcelain crown." That seemed to be the best because gold is safe, right? Wrong.

In 1999, after seeing some patients with heavy-metal health problems, I questioned the type of metal I was using in crowns. I called my dental laboratory and asked Craig, the manager, what percentages of each metal were in the gold and porcelain crowns I was prescribing. (In the US, states require a dental laboratory to fabricate restorations only under the written prescription of a dentist.) This was a *huge* dental laboratory I was using, making hundreds of crowns for dentists.

"Gee, Don, I don't know what the exact metals and percentages are," Craig said. "I'll look them up and call you back."

If Craig didn't know what was in the crowns, no one should assume that their dentist would know what materials they were putting in their patient's mouths.

He called me back. The "gold" metal I thought I had been using was in fact *not* gold—not pure gold, anyway. Platinum is also considered "gold" for the purposes of manufacturing crowns. I knew researchers had not found elemental platinum to pose a health risk in the body, although the jury was still out for organo-platinum compounds, platinum salts and the so-called cis forms used in chemotherapy. I decided to look further into the crown metal issue.

In 1984 the American Dental Association Council on Dental Materials, Instruments and Equipment set up specific dental alloy categories. Four of the categories are regulated and certified by the Identalloy® Council, a non-profit organization. This organization issues certificates with each alloy, listing the metals in the particular alloy along with their percentages.

The alloys are classified into four general groups: high noble (HN), noble (N), predominately base (PB) and cobalt base. Noble metals are gold, platinum and palladium. The classification defines the "noble metal content" as follows:

♦ HN = a noble metal content of 60% or greater and a gold content of 40% or greater

♦ N = a noble metal content of 25% or greater

♦ PB = a noble metal content of less than 25%.

As you can see, this standard classification allows the dentist to tell patients they are getting a gold crown when in reality the "high-noble" alloy, to be so called, requires only 40% gold. There must be at least 60% of gold, platinum and palladium to qualify for the "high

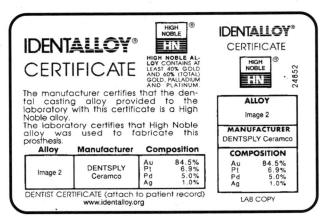

Figure 2-1: This is a "noble" alloy containing mostly palladium, a suspected carcinogen.

noble" alloy. *The balance of the metal alloy can contain anything else.*

The "gold" alloy I was using for so many years is shown in Figure 2-3. It's brand name is Image2® and contains:

♦ 84.5% gold

♦ 6.9% platinum

♦ 5.0% palladium

♦ 1.0% silver

♦ 0.6% unknown metal.

> ...not one of their dentists used pure gold. They all used other metals in the crowns...

I thought I was getting gold or at least gold and platinum alloy but instead I was getting over 6% other metals that were leeching out into my patients' bodies.

I called Craig again. I told him that when I wrote "gold and porcelain" on the prescription slip sent with the patient's case, I thought I was getting 100% gold under the porcelain. He explained the

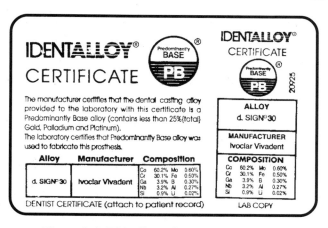

Figure 2-2: This alloy of various metals is predominately "base."

classification system to me and explained that the alloy they used was considered "gold." I told *him* that many of my patients were especially sensitive to restorative materials and had health-related issues. I wanted only pure gold metal under their crowns to prevent reactions to other metals leeching out from the crowns. He told me that his dental laboratory did not even possess pure gold or gold and

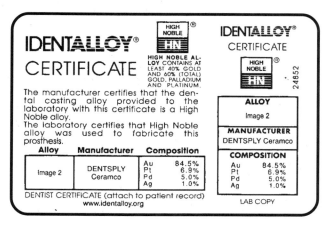

Figure 2-3: This is the alloy I once used: gold and metals, considered a "high noble" alloy.

platinum alloy to use for a crown. In fact, not one of their dentists used pure gold. They all used other metals in the crowns they prescribed.

In the end, the lab had to obtain a special order of an alloy just for me—one that was 100% gold, or rather a gold and platinum alloy, since the platinum was needed for strength. They kept this alloy locked in their lab just for Dr. Robbins' use. The content of this Degudent® G alloy I began using is shown in Figure 2-4.

I was still not confident that the other metals used in crowns were

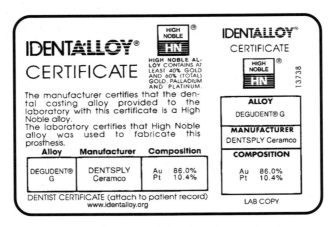

Figure 2-4: The pure gold and platinum alloy I now use.

safe for patients. The majority of my patients with crowns that are all metal or have metal underneath porcelain have bad reactions in their gum tissues surrounding the margins (edges) of the crowns. Over short periods of time (sometimes only six months or a year) the gum would apparently recede more from the metal margin than from a natural tooth surface or a porcelain surface. It is common to see red and swollen inflammation at the margin of the gums around these crowns. (See Figures 2-5 and 2-6, page 112.) In my opinion, this type of reaction contributes to general periodontal disease. And then I realized: *metal in crowns was no longer needed.*

A WOLF IN SHEEP'S CLOTHING

Metal in crowns (not pure gold crowns) exposes patients to metal leakage and possible toxicity. But there are also valid physical dental reasons not to use metal when restoring natural teeth.

The full coverage of the top of a badly decayed or broken down tooth presents two advantages. By covering the whole tooth with a crown, right down to below the gumline, the remaining tooth structure is protected from fracturing and the crown material itself cannot decay. Such coverings are normally made of metal coated in porcelain fused to the metal for strength. However both these advantages of full coverage apply equally well to porcelain restorations made *without* a metal base. In either case, it is the crown porcelain that can break and not the tooth, though fracture of the porcelain is not common if the restoration is done properly.

There are, however, far more serious disadvantages than advantages to using metal to restore the tooth.

1. X-rays cannot penetrate the metal covering on a tooth. Decay can occur and do severe damage to what remains of the tooth underneath before outward signs of a problem are visible. It is quite common to have a patient present in my office with an old crown in their hand that has just fallen off. Upon examination, the remaining tooth is decayed thoroughly, sometimes right to the gumline, and sometimes requiring root canal treatment and a new crown to save it. Sometimes too much decay has occurred, gone on unnoticed for too long, and the tooth is now hopeless and must be extracted.

Porcelain restorations, on the other hand, allow x-rays to pass through so early decay can usually be diagnosed in time to prevent a major disaster.

2. For decades (and even today in some offices) mercury-amalgam filling material was used to build up the inside of a severely decayed tooth. This was necessary to support the full crown that was

made over what was left of the tooth. But the mercury under the gold and metal crown is not stable and is absorbed into the body as soon as it is released.

As we've seen, when two dissimilar metals touch, they can generate a minute electric current that causes the metals to break down faster. This galvanic current can also cause sensitivity or pain for the patient.

As you can see in Figure 2-7 on page 112, it's not usually possible to see this leaking mercury from an examination or an x-ray. In my opinion, where there is a suspicion that mercury may be underneath a crown, that crown should be replaced safely with porcelain-bonded restorations, after the mercury filling has been safely removed.

3. The longevity of a full crown restoration is between five and 20 years. Given that parameter, it is likely that most patients will need to have their crown remade several times during their life, depending, of course, upon how old they are when the first one is done. The drilling off of all the surface tooth structure just to fit an artificial tooth restoration is an extremely destructive procedure. A lot of good tooth structure is usually drilled away. There may not be enough tooth structure remaining to recrown the tooth two or three times. Extraction and tooth replacement (probably with an implant)—a costly procedure—is then the only option.

Porcelain-bonded restorations do not need all the good tooth structure removed, hence more tooth is available to use in the future.

4. Gum tissue does not like to be against or near metal. If a non-biocompatible metal is used for a crown, the gum will recede, inflame and eventually cause periodontal disease and bone recession.

5. Gold and metal crowns do not bond well to a natural tooth. The restoration stays on when it is properly fitted to the drilled tooth and buildup, and cement fills the space between the crown

and the tooth surface to create a mechanical bond. This may sound good. You may be thinking of the advertisement that shows a construction worker hanging from a steel girder by a helmet that's bonded to the beam. But dental cement is not a bonding cement and is nowhere near as strong as that stuff. Over time, *it washes out from the crown and allows saliva, food and bacteria to enter and decay underneath.*

Porcelain-bonded restorations, on the other hand, are not only mechanically cemented onto the tooth but form a chemical bond that seals the space to prevent any intrusion. The bonding resin cement does not wash out from the crown and continues to hold it securely.

6. Metal used under the porcelain on crowns and in other tooth restorations causes cosmetic problems. Most of the population aspires to looking natural and this extends to our teeth. People do not want gold or silver-colored restorations in their teeth that darken the smile. And although porcelain constructed well looks amazingly like a natural tooth, if gold or metal lies underneath, the porcelain will look dull and lifeless. On a front tooth this is particularly unattractive and very noticeable upon smiling. Even worse is the exposed dark margin of the crown when the gum recedes: a black line at the gumline of the crown. Please see Figure 2-8, page 112.

THE TOXIC CROWN

⟨⟨©

Angelina looked like you could knock her over with a feather. She was a tiny 68-year-old woman with a sweet disposition who had consulted with untold numbers of physicians and dentists over the previous four years. She found me through my website and thought a new approach to her problem might help.

"I have a constant burning sensation in my mouth. It gets worse at times but it's almost always there. I've tried everything to get rid of it and my doctors have tried all kinds of medications. Nothing seems to change the burning even a little bit."

I examined her mouth and reviewed some possibilities.

"You have five teeth with mercury amalgam fillings in them. It is possible the mercury or the copper or tin might be affecting you this way. Even if it doesn't change the burning after their removal, you will still be safer by not having the mercury in your mouth."

She agreed and in two weeks we had the fillings replaced by bonded resin. A month later she was back.

"I know they had to come out Dr. Robbins," she told me sadly. "But the burning is no better."

I took another look in her mouth.

"You have four porcelain and metal crowns in your mouth. There is no way to be sure if they have mercury underneath that is leaking out, since the metal blocks the x-rays, but I'd recommend replacing them with porcelain restorations. I've had success with some patients when their complaints were general but their symptoms improved when the metal crowns and any mercury underneath were replaced. I can't guarantee any improvement in the burning but I do know that any metals in the crowns themselves are leeching into your mouth. If you're sensitive to any of them, that could be the cause of your burning sensation."

There were foods Angelina had to avoid and she couldn't rest comfortably with the sensation. The burning was becoming unbearable and affecting her quality of life. She decided to replace the crowns.

By the next month, all four crowns had been replaced with bonded porcelain restorations. Two of the four old crowns had mercury amalgam underneath and decay that was not visible until the crowns were removed. I removed the crowns safely. I called her a few weeks later to see how she was doing and even I was surprised: she was better.

"I'm not getting too excited, Dr. Robbins, but for years I've not been able to use vinegar in my salads because it made the burning worse. Now I've tried it and I can use vinegar without any increase in the burning. The burning is still there but it's less and seems to be going away slowly. I'm so much better and I want to thank you for helping me."

I told her how glad I was to hear she was better. I said I'd see her at her next routine dental checkup.

By then, the burning had become very slight. Angelina was happy and functioning normally.

I've come to understand that toxic exposures from crowns that contain metal (and other metal restorations, such as metal inlays, onlays, partial crowns, etc.) can affect our health. Dental problems such as Angelina's can be caused by nothing more than metal being used in the crown construction—metal most dentists accept without question. Unfortunately, our health can be threatened by the off-gassing of metal vapors that act on the whole body.

> …that toxic exposures from crowns that contain metal (and other metal restorations, such as metal inlays, onlays, partial crowns, etc.) can [adversely] affect our health.

So how do you know if your body will react—negatively—to exposure to a particular metal? The reactions you may have are not usually like those you experience seasonally (e.g., hayfever, grass allergy) or from exposure to penicillin or iodine in shellfish. Instead, the reaction to metals is caused by lymphocytes, white blood cells in your body. There is now a highly sophisticated test to determine if your body is going to react to a particular metal. The MELISA® test not only reveals a potential allergic reaction but discloses whether it will be a slight reaction or a major reaction.

Here's a quick survey of metals that have been used in dental alloys.

Aluminum

Aluminum is an extremely reactive metal and corrodes rapidly when in contact with other metals. When aluminum makes contact with caustic and acidic solutions, it can release dangerous vapors. Inhaling these vapors can causes breathing difficulties, with coughing, shortness of breath and mucosal irritation.

Some studies have linked aluminum to Alzheimer's disease.

Beryllium

Beryllium is a known carcinogen, and is listed as such by the US Center for Disease Control, the US National Institute of Health (NIH), and the US Agency for Toxic Substances and Disease Registry (ATSDR). Dental laboratory personnel who are exposed to larger amounts of beryllium dust and vapors can suffer from acute to chronic exposure, with pneumonia, bronchitis and other lung diseases as a consequence. Beryllium has been used commonly in the metals of crowns.

The chronic exposure patients receive from beryllium in a crown for five to 20 years or more can eventually exert a serious effect on their health. Beryllium attacks the immune system and affects the body's defenses. An estimated 1% to 15% of the population become sensitive to beryllium. Symptoms of chronic exposure include breathing problems, cough, fatigue, chest and joint pain, weight loss and fevers.

Boron

Inhaled boron causes irritation of the nose, throat and eyes, and researchers have linked boron to low sperm counts and birth defects. In general, however, no obvious permanent deleterious effects have been observed as a consequence of low chronic boron exposure.

Copper

Although a trace amount of copper is important for the normal functioning of our metabolism, abnormally high levels give rise to definitive pathology. You'll remember Mark, who had 11 "gold" crowns that were 30% copper. Copper is a component of more than 30 enzymes in the human body. It is involved with collagen synthesis and development of connective tissue, nerve coverings and bone. It's needed for iron and energy metabolism. But high levels of copper may, over time, result in liver and kidney damage, neurological problems and death. People with certain liver diseases and those with an inherited inability to metabolize copper are more at risk.

Iron

Iron becomes a medical problem if there is an inherited genetic disorder, hemochromatosis, that allows too much iron to be absorbed into the body. This condition causes fatigue, weakness, weight loss and stomach and joint pain.

Nickel

Nickel is a known carcinogen, recognized by the International Agency for Research on Cancer (ARC), and can cause sensitization of the skin, and respiratory distress (asthma and pneumonitis).

> Nickel is a known human carcinogen, yet is one of the most common metals used in dental alloys for crowns, dentures and orthodontic wires and brackets.

About 10% to 20% of the population is sensitive to nickel and sensitization can be triggered or increased by skin contact with nickel over periods of time. This will result in more health reactions to the metal, especially as a skin (or mucous membrane) rash. This metal is not indicated for use in crowns since the chronic contact with the tongue, lips and oral tissues can lead to chronic inflammation and irritation. But believe it or not, it still shows up in many crown metals, especially less expensive non-precious alloys.

Molybdenum

The US governmental occupational safety agency, the National Institute for Occupational Safety and Health (NIOSH), determined that although exposure to the insoluble forms of molybdenum metal presents lower toxicity than other forms, there is evidence that respiratory effects result from even this small exposure. The conclusion by Mogilvskaya published in the American Conference of Governmental industrial Hygienists (ACGIH) in 1986 states "the metal and the dioxide proved minimally poisonous."

Tin

Tin, although released from dental amalgam fillings along with mercury and copper, appears to have an innocuous profile. Few adverse health

> My own dental laboratory technician did not know what metals were in the crowns he was making for dentists.

effects have been reported as a result of exposure to tin, either inorganic or oganic.

Lithium

The US Office of Environmental Health Hazard Assessment (OEHHA) considers lithium a serious health concern only when it contacts water to form lithium hydroxide, a strong corrosive base.

Palladium

Palladium may be present in metal crowns in proportions as high as 78.5%. Like mercury, palladium is biomethylated (made organic) in the digestive tract, which makes the metal molecule more toxic than the inorganic form. Being organic, the metal molecule can pass through cell membranes and can cause blocking of enzyme functions.

Lenntech, a water and air filtration group, considers palladium highly toxic and carcinogenic. According to the US Occupational Safety and Health Administration (OSHA) and the American National Standards Institute (ANSI), palladium has caused bone marrow, liver and kidney damage in experimental animals. Other animal experiments indicate that it may interfere with the use of energy by nerves and muscles, induce lung malfunctions, and produce abnormal fetuses.

The conclusion is obvious: there are simply too many potential reactions and too many combinations of metals and too many possible negative health consequences to risk having an untested assortment of metals placed in your mouth for decades. Some of the metals used have unknown health potentials while others are known carcinogens and should never be used. Some metals may pose short-term health threats for susceptible individuals, while others may accumulate over time for long-term health risks. Unless my patients know exactly what metal was used for their crown, I routinely recommend they consider replacement with a non-metallic porcelain restoration. If you're considering the placement of new crowns in your mouth, now is the time to make the safe decision.

3
FLUORIDE

"What responsible health authority would feed a
baby fluoride at 250 times the level that nature
intended, and not even investigate to see if any
damage might have occurred? God provides no
protective veil for such a reckless practice."

Dr. Paul Connett
Professor of Chemistry
St. Lawrence University, NY

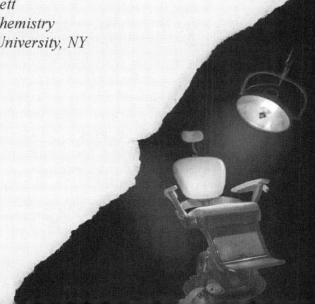

Fluoride, like mercury, is one of the fundamental elements that comprise the physical world. It is number 9 on the periodic table and related to its fellow "halogen" elements: chloride, bromide and iodide. In its pure form, fluoride is a corrosive and poisonous yellowish-brown gas, but it's never found in this form in nature, since fluoride is the most reactive of all the elements and quickly bonds as the ion "fluoride" to other molecules. For this reason, its isolation in the nineteenth century proved exceptionally difficult and exceptionally hazardous. The scientists who died in the attempt are known as the "fluoride martyrs."

> ...few dentists and pediatricians know the exact amount of fluoride that can cause life-threatening events in children.

❧

"Good morning, Dr. Robbins."

I looked down and saw 5-year-old Timmy sitting in my hygienist Susan's dental chair. Boys that age look so cute with their corduroy pants and button-down shirts. Timmy was bright eyed and alert and checking out all the things he could see and touch from the chair. The more familiar the child is with the dentist's tools, the less apprehensive and the more cooperative they become. In my practice, we usually let them hold the air-water syringe and blow a water spray into the sink or feel the suction tube on the skin of their hands so it isn't so scary being in the chair.

"Good Morning. So how's Timmy doing today?"

Mom was sitting on a giant "molar" seat in the hygiene room, showing maternal concern for her son. Her eyebrows were knitted. There was something on her mind.

"He's fine," Mom said. "But we were wondering if we could skip the fluoride treatment for Timmy today?" Mom was uncomfortable, evading my eyes, looking back and forth between Susan and Timmy. Clearly she, like most people, did not like the idea of challenging a doctor's recommendations.

"Is there a problem with Timmy getting the fluoride today?" I asked.

"Well, the last time he was here Susan gave him a fluoride treatment. When we left he said he felt sick and by the time we got home he threw up. I was hoping we could avoid that today."

"I'm sorry Timmy had a bad reaction. You should have called me when you got home to let me know he was sick. I might have suggested something to help. I still don't think it is a good idea to skip his fluoride treatment today. The topical fluoride in the trays goes into the teeth that are already erupted in his mouth. The fluoride goes into the teeth surfaces and protects them against decay. The fluoride supplements I prescribed last time for Timmy to take daily at home go into the teeth that are still developing, to strengthen the actual tooth structure against decay after they erupt.

"Some children swallow a little too much of the fluoride while the trays of fluoride gel are in their mouths. We tell the children to try to not swallow the gel and when we remove the trays we tell them to spit out as much as they can into the sink. I guess Timmy swallowed too much fluoride gel last time and it upset his stomach. If that happens again, just give him some milk or yogurt and that will settle his stomach down. But he is a little older now and understands more, so there's less chance of him swallowing too much fluoride."

Mom nodded but I could tell she was not convinced. Timmy got his fluoride treatment that day anyway.

This scenario was repeated many times during the first few years of my dental practice. Parents would tell me about their child getting sick or nauseous after the treatment and their not wanting to come back because of the "icky" stuff in their mouth. Not a good way to teach children how good it was to have dental checkups.

What I *wasn't* telling Timmy's mom was what dental students are taught in dental school about topical fluoride treatments. They're told to be careful about children swallowing the fluoride because *if a child swallows too much fluoride they can go into a coma or even die.* How many patients do you think were *ever* told that by their dentists? As you will shortly see, few dentists and pediatricians know the exact amount of fluoride that can cause life-threatening events in children. Few even know the official protocol as to why and when fluoride should be used or what contraindications against using fluoride are recommended by the pro-fluoride American Dental Association.

✺

"Mom, where's George?"

Sharon, 14 years old, was munching on a carrot in the kitchen. George was her 5-year-old brother and she hadn't seen him since she got back from school.

Carol was unpacking groceries, getting ready for dinner. "He's upstairs sleeping." She replied. "He didn't feel very good after we got back from the dentist this afternoon. I've been checking on him but he's on his bed sleeping."

Carol had taken George to a checkup appointment early that afternoon. He was examined by the dentist and his teeth were polished by the hygienist. A good patient at five, George got his fluoride treatment without a problem before he left the office. Of course mom had followed the hygienist's instructions and made sure he had nothing to eat or drink for 30 minutes afterwards.

Sharon was getting iced tea out of the refrigerator. "I hated that fluoride stuff when I used to get it. It always made me gag and tasted bad. I always thought I had an upset stomach after the appointment."

"Well, dinner's almost ready. I'll check on him again but he did look a little green when we got home." Carol covered the pot on the stove and went upstairs to George's room. When she peered in, he was stirring on the bed.

"George, dinner's ready. Wash up and come on down.

Sharon set the table so we're ready to go!"

Slowly, George got out of bed. "Okay, mom" was all he could muster.

The rest of the family were seated at the table and starting to eat when George walked into the kitchen. "I don't feel good" he said as he sat at the table.

Before anyone could answer, he vomited all over himself. It was bright blue-colored, foaming liquid and it ran down his shirt. Carol jumped up and examined her son. His color seemed better and he was alert, but crying and clearly upset. Sharon was grossed out and said "See mom! He got sick on that fluoride stuff too!"

Carol saw the blue mess, the same color as the fluoride treatment the hygienist had given him hours earlier.

Too much swallowed fluoride causes a nauseous, sick feeling. The body is telling you this substance is not good for you. It is trying to get it out by vomiting. Isn't it ridiculous to assume that telling a young child not to swallow a solution *in their mouths* will prevent them from doing so? And how can a dentist possibly tell how much of the solution the child has actually swallowed? In cases where too much fluoride is swallowed, *time is critical*. You must stop the swallowed fluoride from being absorbed by the body. The calcium in dairy products will bind the fluoride in the stomach and help prevent absorption. Once absorbed through the stomach lining and into the blood stream, there is no way to effectively remove it before *irreversible* poisoning takes place. Emergency medical care is essential.

Even when I was attending dental school, I was inclined to wonder, since coma or death was a possibility, if maybe dentists should not be using this chemical in *any* patient. After a few years of practice I discontinued recommending or performing fluoride treatments in my office. They are still recommended and performed by most dentists in the country but, as I'm going to show, the truth is this: *fluoride is not safe, is harmful to your health and is not particularly effective as an anti-cavity fighter.*

⚂

It was 8:30 Monday morning and I was about to see a new patient. Monday mornings are never a doctor's friend. You never know what to expect right after the weekend. I have had half my Monday patients cancel their appointments that same morning because they had to work unexpectedly, were ill or found themselves out of town. I have come into the office some Mondays to find the electricity was out and we could not see patients that whole day. If it was snowing—or the weekend forecast even hinted at snow—most of my patients would cancel. This doesn't include the Mondays I would get a telephone call at 7:00 a.m. from one of my staff to tell me they were out sick. So I am not particularly fond of Monday mornings.

Today was no different. My office manager, Patty, cornered me as soon as I entered the back door.

"Your first one is a new patient. Mrs. Siegal brought her 19-year-old daughter Debra in for you to look at. She doesn't like the way Debra's smile looks. She said she wasn't happy with what her old dentist said."

Okay so far. I can give an opinion if that's what Mrs. Siegal wants. However, it's never that simple. A patient coming in to a new dentist with the story that their past dentist wouldn't or couldn't help them, or said something the patient didn't like, that's a red flag. These are usually difficult cases without simple (or cheap) fixes.

I've had women crying in the chair about a dental disaster that happened to them earlier. Some patients are enraged that their old dentist could treat them so badly and do such a lousy job. Most are upset that their previous dentist did not even tell them the truth of what was happening in their mouths. I really hate being the bearer of bad tidings. I don't like being the one to have to tell people bad news. But I tell the patient the truth. I don't sugar-coat it, even if it's the patient's fault. Then I try to help them get through it.

"Good morning. I'm Dr. Robbins, glad to meet you."

I shook the hand of the middle-aged woman sitting in my assistant's chair (my assistant's chair—my assistant was standing!) whom I assumed to be Mrs. Siegal. She was well dressed, with modest makeup and medium-length brown hair brushed back off her face, as if she was going to a business meeting.

"Hello," she said, shaking my hand and exhibiting a comfortable manner of command. "I'm Debra's mother, Joanne. This is Debra."

She nodded to the attractive young redhead in the dental chair.

"We have a problem we hope you can help us with."

I turned my attention to Debra and shook her hand. She was a naturally beautiful girl with hazel eyes and minimal makeup, but only a half smile. I smiled.

"Hello Debra. What seems to be the problem?"

Mom chimed in before Debra could speak. "She doesn't like the way her teeth look and she doesn't smile enough,"

Oh oh. When the parent speaks for the older child (or for the spouse) there can be difficulty understanding exactly what concerns the parent and what concerns the patient. The two worries may be completely different or can be the same.

I tried again.

"Debra what don't *you* like about your teeth?"

"I have these white spots on my front teeth," Debra answered before her mother. "They're really bad and show when I smile."

She still wasn't smiling.

"She's studying the theater in school," Mom hurried to re-enter the conversation. "A couple of her teachers remarked that her teeth needed some work if she wanted to succeed in acting. Our dentist told us there wasn't much he could do short of placing full porcelain veneers or crowns on 10 of her upper teeth. I thought there might be another way so I came here."

I set up to examine her teeth and took a look.

"I don't understand how this could happen!" Mrs. Siegal

exclaimed. "My husband and I took our children to the dentist religiously every six months. We did whatever was needed and—look!—she has these damaged-looking teeth!"

Sure enough, there were large and unattractive white and brown blotches and spots over most of Debra's front teeth. I had seen hundreds of cases like this and immediately knew the cause and the limited solutions. I hated being the bearer of bad news but had no choice—again.

"I'm afraid what we're looking at is dental fluorosis. It's caused by overexposure to fluoride during the years the teeth were forming, anytime between age two and 12. Was Debra taking any fluoride as a child? Was your public water fluoridated or did you have well water?" I asked.

Mrs. Siegal became agitated. "We have fluoridated public water. She has been drinking that water her whole life. We *all* have. Her pediatrician recommended she take chewable fluoride tablets as a supplement when she was little to prevent cavities. Her dentist agreed. She took fluoride tablets until she was 10."

I had to explain.

"The fluoride tablets weren't needed for Debra because of the fluoride she was getting in her drinking water. In fact the fluoride in her drinking water wasn't needed either. It's generally recognized nowadays that children are exposed to fluoride all over in their diet. Supplemental fluoride only causes overexposure. This white staining is permanent damage from the excess fluoride."

Mrs. Siegal exploded.

"You mean to tell me they had me give pills to Debra that caused this ugly stain on her teeth? They never said anything about the possibility of them causing permanent damage to the teeth! Why didn't our dentist tell us what was happening?"

"Most dentists were taught in dental school how to prescribe fluoride supplements. Although the US Food and Drug Administration (FDA) and the US Academy of Pediatric Medicine changed the rules years ago and cautioned doctors to evaluate more carefully and fully who should get these supplements, many dentists blindly prescribe them anyway. This staining is actually the earliest visible sign of general fluorosis. There may or may not be other changes in Debra's body from the fluoride overdose."

Mrs. Siegal was digesting what I had said. Finally she sighed and said "What can we do now?"

"Unfortunately the only remedy for stains like these is to construct partial coverage porcelain veneers for the front 10 teeth. They will cover the front stains on her teeth and give her a beautiful smile. The cost will be about $9,000."

They were both stunned, speechless.

ॐ

This situation is quite common in dental offices across the United States and Canada. Dentists and pediatricians prescribe fluoride supplements without understanding the cautions inherent in the product information and federal guidelines themselves. A little further on, we're going to look at the studies that support the proposal that fluoride supplements are being prescribed incorrectly and without proper diagnostic evaluation. In fact there is no reason to ever prescribe fluoride supplements nor to fluoridate public drinking water. The United State is the *only* country to add fluoride to a child's diet.

FLUORIDE AND ME

In my first few years of practice, the late '70s and early '80s, I observed something disturbing in the teeth of teenage patients and young adults who were coming into my office for routine dental checkups. Many had white, chalky stains and/or yellow or brown blotches on their teeth, more often on their front teeth, incisors, canines and premolars. This unattractive discoloration varied in intensity, some patients having very slight white lines on their central or lateral incisor teeth. Many others had most of their tooth surfaces, front and back teeth, covered with high levels of white, yellow and brown. Many patients were self-conscious about how unsightly their teeth looked and would not show a wide smile or consciously expose their teeth while talking. When pressed, they complained about how terrible their teeth looked.

I soon diagnosed the problem as dental fluorosis, a condition caused by ingestion of excess fluoride during the time the teeth were developing. The fluoride actually interferes with the orderly, crystalline formation of the enamel in developing teeth before they erupt into the mouth. The stains and blotches are defective enamel tooth structure that reflects light badly and causes rough and bumpy surfaces on the teeth, making them look horrible. My patients' histories revealed that almost all had been on daily fluoride supplements, fluoride treatments and/or drank fluoridated water as young growing children. I realized that the daily supplemental fluoride tablets that dentists and physicians were prescribing for children, when added to other fluoride sources the child was probably exposed to, were actually supplying excessive fluoride to the body. These supplements had been recommended by the American Dental Association, the US Food and Drug Administration and the supplement manufacturers since the 1950s. They were to be given to *all* children, from liquid fluoride drops after birth through tablets into the early teenage years. When I saw this effect later in their lives, when these patients were in my dental chair, I immediately cut the recommended dosages in half when prescribing the supplements for my child patients.

In the early '80s, I began searching for and reading scientific and toxicology literature about the effects of fluoride. I did not look at the recommendations made by the American Dental Association because they did *not* present a fair and balanced opinion. As far as I was aware, no article on fluoride toxicology warning of the dangers of fluoride, either cosmetically or systemically in the body and bones, ever appeared in the ADA journal. More astonishingly, I realized that, since the '50s, *the ADA has had a financial interest in the success of fluoride.*

You've probably observed the following yourself but never realized its significance. When you go into a drug store and walk down the aisle for medications such as an aspirin or antihistamine, or the aisle with antacids on the shelves, you see many products in various packaging. But if you look at the box or tube, you see no mention of the American Medical Association. Now take a walk down the aisle with the dental products on the shelves. Pick up any name-brand toothpaste or floss and look at the label. It says. "Seal of Approval of the American Dental Association." Now consider this: *companies must pay to have their product "evaluated" and use of this seal must be approved by the ADA.* Only then may the "official" seal be placed on their products. The ADA collects huge sums of money each year, directly and indirectly, from the use of this official seal. The association cannot claim to be objective evaluators for the protection of the public because it has a vested interest in the sale of these "approved" products. This also motivates big corporations with products used for oral hygiene to advertise that fact and make it seem as though their products have a special advantage over their competitor's products. The public spends billions of dollars each year on toothpaste, floss, mouth rinses and other oral products. The ADA seal is a big advantage that fluoride and other approved products have over natural products that are also available, may be safer and do an excellent job. The product developers and manufacturers have a *vested interest in maintaining the status quo of the ADA seal and would probably lose sales if the seal was eliminated.*

This is important to remember: the ADA is a trade organization very much like the Teamsters or teacher's unions. Its officers and managers are looking out for the interests of their members, not the health of the general public. There is nothing wrong with a trade group promoting the interests of their members *unless they attempt to disguise themselves as public health advocates.* When the government or corporations consult with them on matters of national dental health or the safety of dental products, the ADA has a duty to help their membership get what they want for their practices, regardless of the consequences for the public. Clearly, government should be consulting with independent scientific investigators and universities that perform independent research and who have no financial or political interests in the outcomes of their studies. It is no different than buying a car. If you want objective comparisons between automobile manufacturers, would you ask the Ford or Nissan dealership which car is better? Would you not go to an independent automobile magazine or website that lists all the alternative choices and so allows a legitimate comparison?

And this little-known fact is worth considering: the ADA has experienced declining membership over the last few decades. At last estimate, less than 60% of dentists belong to their organization. Shouldn't we consider listening to the opinions of the other 40% of dentists?

In my review of the literature, there were plenty of medical references and studies supporting the view that fluoride was not only damaging to tooth development but, if swallowed, dangerous to the rest of the body for child or adult alike, but especially for children. By the end of the '80s I stopped prescribing all fluoride supplements for children. When a child was in my office, I asked the parents if they were giving their child daily fluoride supplements as prescribed by their physician or previous dentist. If the child was taking the supplement, I recommended stopping its use and told the parents about the dangers, with excess fluoride use, of damaged teeth and possible bone changes.

Indeed, by the late '90s, more and more scientific research was emerging that showed damage to teeth from ingested fluoride. This was no longer a "cosmetic" problem as originally labeled by the FDA. The new studies were showing that the tooth surfaces are actually weakened and damaged by the chemical. It is also now known that ingested fluoride is a more serious threat to one's overall health than ever suspected.

FLUOROGATE

What follows is a tale of intrigue, deceit and conspiracy. I'm not recounting it with pleasure or to frighten my readers. It's simply the truth. The origin of fluoride use in the United States is a textbook example of government cover-up, legal manipulation and denial of responsibility.

The public unraveling of this story began in 1997, when the *Christian Science Monitor* commissioned two investigators to establish the truth about fluoride: that fluoride was a safe, dental-decay preventative. They never dreamed they'd turn up information long buried under a cloak of US government security, a cloak that had begun to fall away as government documents were declassified and released in the mid-1990s. After almost a year of uncovering information and searching for supporting documentation, the principal *Monitor* investigators, Chris Bryson and Joel Griffiths, presented the paper's editors with the whole twisted story. The publisher decided it was far too controversial at that time and decided not to publish it. But in view of the widespread belief in fluoride's efficacy and its general popularity in the United States, and realizing the implications for the government, and more importantly the safety and health of the public at large, the authors gave the story to various public forums to publish as they wished.

So gather round, dear readers, and perhaps toast a comforting marshmallow or two. Dr. Robbins is going to tell you a really scary campfire story.

The first person to go on record as noticing damage to teeth from fluoride was Dr. Frederick McKay, in 1901 in Colorado Springs, Colorado. Dr. McKay observed the unusual permanent stains on the teeth of local residents and called it "mottled enamel." The residents in the area were quite aware of the stained teeth; *they* called it "Colorado brown stain." Dr. McKay concluded that something in the public water supply was responsible for the tooth damage and he hypothesized that the same agent was responsible for the decreased tooth decay he observed in local residents.

In 1909, a deep well was dug in Bauxite, Arkansas for a public water supply. Some time afterwards, Dr. F. L. Robertson, an area dentist, noted "mottled tooth enamel" appearing on the teeth of local children. The deep well was the suspected cause of the aberration and in 1927 Bauxite abandoned it as a source of water. Through newly developed spectrographic analysis, it was determined in 1930 that the water from the well contained high concentrations of fluoride: 13.7 ppm. Back in Colorado, this new analysis method inspired Dr. McKay to send samples of his area's water for analysis. Those local samples demonstrated that high fluoride levels—between 2.0 and 12.0 ppm—were causing the damaged enamel in local children.

Yet, though fluoride concentrations of 2.0 ppm had by now been shown to cause damage to children's teeth, the National Institute of Health encouraged the testing of residents in four US cities by adding "negligible" levels of fluoride to their water—generally from 1.0 to 1.2 ppm. These studies began in 1945 and ran 13 to 15 years.

How, given what was already known, could this meddling "experiment" ever come to be carried out?

During World War II, as the US hastened to develop more effective weapons, the development of the atomic bomb—the famous Manhattan Project—was a central though secret initiative. One of the main research and development facilities of the Manhattan Project was in southern New Jersey, in the heart of prosperous farmland. An A.E.I. duPont du Nemours Company chemical factory was located here, in the town of Deepwater, and during the course of the war, the factory turned out tens of thousands of pounds of fluoride to be used in the production of weapons-grade plutonium and uranium.

In the 1940s, there was no US Occupational Safety and Hazard Administration or other worker-protection agencies. Workers in the DuPont plants were grossly exposed to all kinds of toxic substances and dangerous working conditions. Fluoride was one of the most dangerously toxic yet little known of these chemicals and its concentration in the work areas was extraordinarily high. The reports on fluoride production in the plant, revealed in hundreds of once-secret declassified documents 50 years later, tell us that the workers had to wear rubber boots because the fluoride was eating through the nails in their shoes. There were no protective gear or breathing systems to protect the men from toxic fumes. The classified version of a 1948 fluoride-safety report revealed that most of the men had no teeth left as a consequence of the fluoride levels. The official, released version stated truthfully enough that *they had fewer cavities*. Conditions were so severe that workers died from this fluoride exposure, usually from contact with and/or breathing in of the toxic fumes. In fact, after the war, the first lawsuits against the United States government for wrongful deaths related to the Manhattan Project were not, as one might think, those claiming exposure to radioactivity. The suits were filed to redress deaths from fluoride exposure. After the end of WWII, this lethal exposure to fluoride in the course of plutonium and uranium production continued through the Cold War. It appears to have been ignored as an issue of national security.

Precautions against leakage of fluoride from the DuPont facility to the outside southern New Jersey environment through water and air were inadequate to say the least. Indeed they were not even seriously considered during planning of the research facility. In 1944 a severe leak vented an enormous amount of fluoride into the air. Within a short time the surrounding farms downwind from the plant, in Salem and Gloucester counties, were to experience the effect, though they could not know the cause. Crops, especially the peach crop, withered and died. Cattle and livestock could not walk or eat. The farmers and families suffered serious health problems sometimes leading to their deaths.

This did not go unnoticed by the government, but instead of rising to the occasion by protecting and treating the surrounding communities, those in charge were concerned about the thousands of potential lawsuits against the government for damage to life and property from the "incidental" fluoride exposure. There was an unseemly scramble to cover up responsibility. Members of the US Atomic Energy Commission, army officers in charge of the project, key Manhattan Project research personnel and government lawyers would meet regularly in secret talks to find a way to divert the cause of the "sickness" away from the fluoride production facility.

The head project investigator, David Ast, met secretly with Harold Hodge, chief pharmacologist for the Manhattan Project, on several occasions between 1944 and 1946. The deception was comprehensive. Even Dr. Hodge's title of pharmacologist was a cover for his real position, which was chief of fluoride toxicity studies for the Manhattan Project. These discussions revolved around *not* releasing any information about the fluoride exposure to surrounding communities and trying to make fluoride and the production plant appear to be uninvolved with the environmental disaster in the area. To put it modestly, David Ast was not an objective investigator. The group kept a tight lid on information about chemical uses and leakage. Meanwhile, when requested by local attorneys, politicians, news services and the local ailing population to reveal how much fluoride was being handled by DuPont in the Deepwater facility, they stonewalled all attempts to force disclosure by refusing to divulge any information in "the interest of national security."

The conspirators decided something more supportive, something truly compelling, was required if they were to truly look like good guys. Someone suggested that a clincher would be to paint fluoride as a "good thing" instead of a toxic killer. And as it turned out, they did just that, with success that must have gone beyond their wildest imaginings.

How it was achieved is a story of breathtaking duplicity.

As we've seen, public health officials in the Midwest such as Dr. McKay had been observing communities where decay rates in the teeth of the local population were low but accompanied by permanent discoloration and staining of teeth. Further investigation had shown naturally high levels of fluoride in the groundwater.

Officials of the Manhattan Project and other government agencies now jumped at what they saw as a remarkable opportunity. If they could show that fluoride was a good decay-preventive chemical, any lawsuits based on the lethal effects of fluoride could be dismissed as unfounded by the courts. The US Public Health Service (many of whose members were involved with the Manhattan Project and the subsequent fluoride cover-up) set out to devise a "scientific study" that would evaluate the effect of fluoridated water on children's teeth. Safety studies would be conducted by the University of Rochester, by the same investigating facility that was to knowingly inject unsuspecting hospital patients with toxic doses of radioactive plutonium as part of notorious human radiation experiments during the Cold War. Many faculty at Rochester were in fact senior bomb-program scientists, including Stafford Warren, the top medical officer of the Manhattan Project, and Harold Hodge.

The now famous Newburgh-Kingston New York study of 1945 to 1956 was underway. In this study, Newburgh, New York had its water fluoridated in 1945 at 1 ppm while Kingston, New York had no fluoride added to their water. The children in each city were evaluated initially for the number of decayed, missing and filled teeth (DMF) in their mouths. The DMF is a common and simple observation-based measure that can assess how dentally challenged a child has been. At the end of the specified time for the study, 10 years, the children in each city would again be evaluated to determine their DMF. The study concluded that the Kingston children had more decay than the Newburgh children. The resulting recommendation from the investigators was that fluoride should be added to community drinking water to help reduce dental decay.

During the study, former Manhattan Project "pharmacologist" Hodge was named to head up the secret Program F that this core group ran behind the very public fluoride study. The group covertly gathered and analyzed the blood and tissue samples from the citizens of Newburgh and Kingston who participated in the public health study. These subjects had no idea that their tissue samples were being analyzed for anything other than to investigate whether fluoride was safe and effective. Program F—carried out with the cooperation of the state health department—was not for purposes of true research and was not conducted by true public health investigators. Like the Kingston-Newburgh study itself, its purpose was to provide legal ammunition in the face of the many lawsuits against the government for bodily injury and wrongful death from fluoride exposure. The investigation was conducted by the defendants. And like the Kingston-Newburgh study, the results were determined beforehand. To this day, all safety reports or evidence of adverse health effects of fluoride use in the study population are missing from the files.

These A-bomb program "researchers" actually played a leading role in the design and implementation of the Newburgh-Kingston study. People such as Henry Barnett, a captain in the Manhattan Project's Medical Section, and John Fertig, with the office of Scientific Research and Development, Pentagon Group, were typical. Hodge considered it was his purpose "to supply evidence useful in the litigation arising from an alleged loss of fruit crop several years ago." He acknowledged that there was an increased blood fluoride level in the human residents in the area but did nothing to help them medically or stop the obstruction of justice. An additional clandestine goal of Program F's Newburgh-Kingston study was to discover any long-term effects of fluoride exposure that might have a useful military application. That was the motivation behind the secret blood and placental tissue evaluations on the unwitting residents. These tissue samples were analyzed by Program F members at the University of Rochester for any possible toxic effects of fluoride and the results of *those* analyses are also still missing.

Thanks to Harold Hodge and the US government, the actual statistical results of the Newburgh–Kingston study were not released at that time to the public or outside scientific community. Only its conclusions were published and promoted. The Program-F scientists published a 1948 study—the one that blithely noted the decline in tooth decay among DuPont workers—in the *Journal of the American Dental Association*. The original version, which showed evidence of severe adverse health effects from fluoride, was censored by the Atomic Energy Commission "for reasons of national security." The published summaries were doctored to reflect the total safety and efficacy of fluoride when used to prevent decay.

Only after 50 years have the results of the Newburgh-Kingston study been made available and the data evaluated properly. Documentation and private letters now reveal the unscientific, illogical and scattered nature of these studies that were specifically designed to showcase fluoride as an effective decay preventive agent. The new evidence reveals tremendous flaws in the method employed during evaluations for the study, and the questionable cover-ups in the interpretation of the data. The method by which the children were evaluated did not include other factors—quality of oral hygiene practiced, other sources of ingested or exposure to fluoride, routine dental visits during the study period, and much else—that could have affected the study results and changed its conclusions, conclusions drawn so many years ago to encourage the fluoridation of the public water supply—and now discredited entirely.

The Newburgh-Kingston paired study—or rather the study's "analysis" showing reduced tooth decay in children—has been held up for generations as prime proof of the effectiveness of fluoride. The general public took up the fluoride cause in an almost emotional response. Everybody wants good-looking teeth. Nobody wants decay or gum disease. An interesting study has shown that others view individuals with visible tooth decay in terms that are not directly related to teeth. They're assumed to be less desirable based on sociability, reliability and cleanliness. The proposition that this fluoride "magic pill" could stop decay was compelling. People wanted to believe.

Dr. Henry Trendley Dean, a dentist, has been lauded for "discovering" that 1 ppm of fluoride is an effective dilution for water fluoridation. The ADA lists him as one of the great achievers in dentistry. The International Association for Dental Research (IADR) elected him president from 1944 to 1945 and since has offered an annual award in his name—The H. Trendley Dean Memorial Award—for distinguished accomplishments in research and development in the fields of behavioral science, epidemiology and public health. In reality, he appears to have been an honest dentist who questioned the use of fluoride for fighting tooth decay right from the beginning. After his 1932 examination of children with mottled teeth in Minonk, Illinois, he wrote the Surgeon General of his findings and concerns. He wondered if mottled teeth might be an oral manifestation of a general toxicity. The hair of some of the Illinois children was unusually coarse, like horse hair. Their fingernails were not normal. Physicians in the area noted large numbers of skin disorders among those drinking the city water supply. Dr. Dean wrote that there would be a follow-up investigation of this disturbing evidence, but there never was one. In fact, during a meeting of the Newburgh Fluoridation Study Committee in April 1944—part of the planning of the city fluoride studies—Dr. Dean himself testified about fluoride's adverse effects. He stated that the population examined by the United States Public Health Service in Texas communities that had high fluoride levels in their drinking water, showed marked health changes including

♦ Severe bony changes in the lumbar and pelvis

♦ Changes in the long bone thicknesses that pushed out marrow spaces, causing reduced hemoglobin production

♦ Increased cataracts

♦ Structural changes in the nails.

He "could not agree," he said, "that the proposed program could be considered a perfectly safe procedure from a public health point of view." And by a bitter irony, this man was elevated as a hero of fluoridation.

Regardless of all the political maneuvering, some simple facts remain, facts ignored by almost every practicing dentist in the United States, facts that the American Dental Association does not acknowledge, facts that the CDC has purposely never investigated:

> Through all the fluoride studies, no safety studies were ever
> fully performed before, during or afterwards. No evaluations
> were ever made of the impact of fluoride on pregnant women,
> nursing mothers, adults and the elderly who also drank the
> fluoridated water. No study was done of the long-term effects
> of ingesting fluoride.[1]

Many people attempted to expose the inadequacies of the fluoridation studies but none was successful. In 1952, during hearings before the House of Representatives, the point was raised by Representative A. L. Miller of Nebraska that there were still no studies on possible deleterious effects of fluoridation on pregnant woman, on old people, and on those with chronic diseases. Not one of the organizations—the American Medical Association, the National Re-

---

[1] Peter Meiers. *The History of Fluorine, Fluoride and Fluoridation. Questionable Fluoride Safety Studies: Bartlett vs. Cameron & Newburgh vs. Kingston*

search Council, the American Public Health Association, or any of the others that testified to the safety of fluoride—had ever carried out any experimental studies or examinations to support their position. He continued "So why would they endorse it when there have been no experiments in that field? That is what bothers me."

Fluoridation: The "Official" Levels

In 1975 the US Environmental Protection Agency (EPA) established the standard Maximum Contaminant Level Goal (MCLG) for fluoride in public drinking water. It was based on an investigative report by scientists reviewing data on fluoride toxicity effects. The MCLG is the level below which there is no known or expected risk to health. Establishing this level is one mandate of the EPA established to protect the public. The scientists and the EPA agreed upon a MCLG of 1.4 to 2.4 ppm (parts per million), the actual concentration depending upon the average temperature of the community to be fluoridated. (Higher temperatures naturally tended to dissolve more fluoride in the water, lower temperatures less.) They considered the dental fluorosis effect "cosmetic" and not adverse to a person's overall health.

Almost immediately after the level was set, individual states started lobbying and complaining about the lower threshold of the permitted maximum level. The regulation *required* each state to conform to the standard but communities in many states had levels that were naturally above allowed maximums. Such states or communities might have had to implement costly devices to *lower* the levels of fluoride in drinking water. South Carolina was especially argumentative, requesting a higher level of 4 ppm be set to allow compliance with the regulations in the many areas of their state that were naturally elevated. Meanwhile, the EPA scientific members were asking for a *decrease* in levels to 1 ppm because of the damage to teeth. Every non-dental group of experts now regarded dental fluorosis as an *adverse health effect*. It was widely considered an early indicator of a

FLUORIDE PRESS RELEASE

The Office of Drinking Water in conjunction with OMB proudly presents their new and improved FLUORIDE REGULATION or "How We Stoped Worrying and Learned to Love Funky Teeth". Up to now EPA, under the Safe Drinking Water Act, has regulated fluoride in order to prevent children from having teeth which looked like they had been chewing brown shoe polish and rocks. The old standard which was based upon the consumer's average shoe size and the phase of the moon, generally kept fluoride levels below 2.4 mg/L. EPA in response to new studies, which only confirmed the old studies, and some flat out political preasure, has decided to raise the standard to 4 mg/L. This increase will allow 40% of all children to have teeth gross enough to gag a maggot. EPA selected this level based upon a cost effectiveness study which showed that it is cheaper for people to keep their mouths shut then to remove the fluoride.

Figure 3-1: Mock press release by EPA scientists to fight political health decisions in 1985

toxic body-burden of fluoride.

During this battle between the EPA scientific group and the EPA politicians, an office memo (see Figure 3-1) was circulated by EPA science workers that mocked management's plan to allow higher than safe levels of fluoride. And indeed, in 1985 the updated drinking water standard was passed. The Maximum Contaminant Level Goal for fluoride had been raised to 4 ppm. About the same time, the condition called "moderate to severe dental fluorosis" was classified as a non-health effect. The damaged teeth were considered a strictly "cosmetic effect." This ruling has not changed since 1985, even though adverse health effects from fluoride have now been documented in new scientific literature for years.

What's in a Label?

Being a typical government bureaucracy, the FDA regulates the allowable range of fluoride concentration in bottled water.

If the water is naturally fluoridated—that is, if the supplier bottles it exactly as it comes out of the ground—the FDA does not require a label stating its fluoride content. If on the other hand the supplier adds any fluoride to the water before it is bottled, the FDA *does* require the total fluoride content to be listed on the label.

This means you can't really know how much fluoride is in the bottle if it is naturally bottled. A supplier could be selling high natural fluoride in the water bottled in one state while the same supplier might sell water in another state bottled from a different source and containing a different level of fluoride. To make matters worse, the FDA regulations show that the allowable natural fluoride levels are *higher than those a supplier is permitted to add to their water*. The general public can buy "natural bottled water" with fluoride levels up to 2.4 ppm and *not be able to tell from the label how much is in there or at what levels.*

> The amount of fluoride in bottled water is not listed on the label (unless the supplier adds *more* fluoride to the water).

I am indebted to the Fluoride Action Network for bringing to my attention the product cited in their notice, below. Fluoridated baby water is a dramatic example of disregard for scientific research and demonstrates how readily children can be exposed to the dangers to over-fluoridation. This water is marketed for *babies* use and was even discouraged by the American Dental Association as a hazard for infants. (http://www.ipetitions.com/petition/walmart/).

TABLE 3. U.S. Food and Drug Administration (FDA) fluoride requirements for bottled water packaged in the United States		
	Maximum fluoride concentration (mg/L) allowed in bottled water	
Annual average of maximum daily air temperature (F) where the bottled water is sold at retail	No fluoride addedto bottled water	Fluoride added to bottled water
53.7	2.4	1.7
53.8-58.3	2.2	1.5
58.4-63.6	2	1.3
63.9-70.6	1.8	1.2
70.7-79.2	1.6	1
79.3-90.5	1.4	0.8

Table 3-1: Fluoride in Bottled Water

Note: FDA regulations require that fluoride be listed on the label only if the bottler adds fluoride during processing; the bottler is not required to list the fluoride concentration, which might or might not be optimal. FDA does not allow imported bottled water with no *added* fluoride to contain >1.4 mg fluoride/L or imported bottled water with added fluoride to contain >0.8 mg fluoride/L.

Source: US Department of Health and Human Services, Food and Drug Administration. 21 CFR Part 165.110. Bottled water. Federal Register 1995;60:57124-30.

The Battle Continues

The ripples of the Manhattan Project continue to effect lives today. Communities in most countries never adopted fluoridation, others have abandoned it, others are still struggling. Calgary, Alberta has had an ongoing debate over fluoridation of their public drinking water for years. There have been threats of lawsuits by parents of children with damaged teeth if the government does not remove the fluoride from the water. Yet today, $2/3$ of the public water supplies in the United States remain fluoridated.

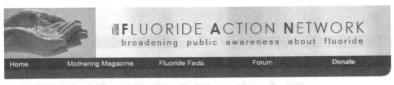

Ask Wal-Mart to Stop Selling Fluoride "Nursery Water" to Infants

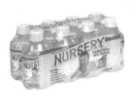

On November 9th, 2006, the American Dental Association (ADA) issued an alert advising parents to avoid fluoridated water when reconstituting infant formula. ADA's advice, however, has been mostly ignored by the media.

Nursery Water, the nation's leading fluoridated water for babies, still markets its product nationwide at Wal-Mart and other major retailers.

Figure 3-2: Infant water marketed with fluoride

At the end of this sorry and frightening tale, you might be wondering about the lawsuits against the government that followed the suffering and deaths of those who worked in the DuPont facility contracted as part of the Manhattan Project.

The University of Rochester team that conducted these tests—and the subsequent cover-ups performed in the name of "national security"—deemed fluoride to be safe. The New Jersey crop and livestock damage and the personal injury lawsuits were dismissed and none of the victims ever received remuneration or even recognition for what had been inflicted upon them.

> Drinking tap water can be hazardous to your health.

FLUORIDE TOXICITY: YOUR TEETH

By this point, I don't need to tell you that fluoride is poisonous to humans. But what is the nature of that toxicity? What effect does it have when there isn't enough of it to dissolve the nails from our shoes? Let me start with our teeth, those useful features that most concern dentists and that have been made to carry responsibility for the introduction of so much fluoride into our lives.

Developing Teeth

During those years when the permanent teeth are developing, roughly between years one to 11, the level of fluoride in a child's body can have a profound effect on how enamel and dentin are produced in the teeth. Since water fluoridation began in the 1950s, it was assumed that only high levels of ingested fluoride during tooth development would cause clinically severe damage to enamel and dentin. It was never stated or proven, however, what constituted a "high level." Tests that might have determined the safety and other effects of fluoride on the teeth, brain and body of children and adults were specifically avoided by governmental agencies trying to promote fluoride usage.

Then, 20 years ago, members of the scientific and medical community began questioning the levels of fluoride recommended for tooth-decay prevention and the effects fluoride might have on other systems of the body. It was reasoned that if an agent could profoundly alter mineral deposition in the teeth of developing children—fluoride bonds very strongly to calcium and prevents it from being utilized elsewhere—it would also have effects on other systems that employ calcium mineralization. Scientific articles in peer reviewed journals began to address these concerns. Overall, they showed that increased fluoride levels in tooth enamel supplant normal calcium levels in the tooth, thereby causing the development of enamel that is not as hard or strong.

How the Damage Is Done

We now know that fluoride interferes with the normal mineralization of enamel and dentin substrate. As the tooth develops, an organic substrate is laid down, a blueprint of the future tooth form. This tooth matrix, made up of amelogenin proteins, is where minerals are deposited in a crystalline pattern. This process allows for smooth, hard and solid enamel surfaces and normal dentin structure. The main mineralization is composed of microcrystalline hydroxyapatite, a biologic form of calcium. As the mineral crystals are organized and deposited, the organic matrix is removed by the body.

If fluoride is present, it causes retention of these soft amelogenin proteins, which interfere with the orderly production of enamel and dentin, causing increased porosity of the enamel surface of the tooth—so-called hypocalcification or hypomineralization—that appears as white spots, lines or discolored regions on the tooth surface. In more extreme cases, the teeth may be deformed or have large brownish areas of damaged structure. These areas of reduced calcium are areas of reduced hardness, with microscopic openings in the actual tooth surface that allow bacteria to colonize and produce acids that in turn lead to decay. The rough surface is also a magnet for stain and plaque accumulation. And, of course, even in mild cases the cosmetic appearance of a person's smile is permanently affected. Repair or replacement of these damaged teeth or tooth surfaces means costly dental treatment. Mrs. Siegal's daughter Debra was a sad example.

Fluoride and Sensitive Teeth: More a Cause than a Cure

The damaging and altering of the structure of dentin as an effect of fluoride also causes abnormal *enlargement* of dentinal tubules that are normally present in the dentin. These adverse effects of fluoride specifically on the dentin of the tooth were noted as early as 1936. As we've seen, fluoride does this by delaying the mineralization of the dentin protein substrate, allowing less calcification of the dentin itself. The larger tubules that result are believed to cause teeth to be more sensitive to normal environmental stimuli such as cold, heat and pressure. This may account for the wide range of sensitivity and pain patients report while having their teeth treated at the dentist's office.

Fluoride: Simply Not Effective

In a 1998 study, the New York State Department of Health compiled data from the same two cities—Newburgh and Kingston, New York—over 50 years after the original study had been used to justify widespread fluoridation. These studies and report were published by dentists Kumar and Green in the *New York State Dental Journal*, February, 1998. Newburgh has been fluoridated since the time of the first study; Kingston has remained unfluoridated. The results of this new study—one of many—show the children of fluoridated Newburgh to have more decay and more discolored teeth (dental fluorosis) than the children of Kingston.

The topical application of fluoride to prevent decay is also in retreat. Though it does prevent acid production by bacteria and therefore prevents tooth decay, it's effective only during the short time it is on the tooth surface. It is quickly washed out of the oral environment by saliva, foods and liquids. There are no long-term preventive effects and topical fluoride certainly does nothing to prevent decay when ingested in any form during development of the teeth.

The past-president of the Canadian Association for Dental Research, Dr. Hardy Limeback, notes that "new research shows that swallowed fluoride carries little, if any, benefit" and continues: "Fluoride's enamel-strengthening effects are primarily topical, or when fluoride touches the outside of the tooth."

> There are no long-term preventive effects and topical fluoride certainly does nothing to prevent decay when ingested in any form during development of the teeth.

Occasionally, solutions containing fluoride are recommended to irrigate periodontal (gum) pockets for patients with peridontitis (gum disease). This is usually performed by the hygienist or dentist during a deep scaling, removing tartar and calculus from under the gums. I recently read a case report of necrosis and permanent loss of bone that illustrates how fluoride can be injurious when applied directly to the soft gum tissue.

We are forced to accept that the recommendation of fluoride for these indications was politically motivated. Sad to say, political forces can still control the findings of unbiased scientific study by putting their own unique spin on the press releases. Organized groups of individuals are petitioning authorities on issues of toxicity and health that have been politically manipulated with the support of big business. After 50 years, government agencies are at last starting to question the safety of some of the dental products and materials they once grandfathered into use. Grandfathering of a product used in health care refers to the approval (by the FDA) of a product for marketing to the public, based on a review of data collected during long-term use of a product by the general public *and* low frequency of side effects reported to state or government health agencies during the use of the product. For a product that is grandfathered into use, it is possible that the high quality clinical studies required for new products undergoing development and approval by the FDA would not be required. (So far this author has uncovered no studies for short- or long-term health effects and adverse events from fluoride ingestion that were ever published.)

For years the FDA has considered dental-amalgam mercury fillings a "device" which has allowed it to avoid peer-reviewed safety studies and reports of adverse health events. Through political efforts mercury has been allowed to be placed in the mouth without restraint.

Meanwhile, just as in Kingston-Newburgh, new studies are constantly being published that refute the efficacy of fluoride as a tooth-decay preventative agent. Unfortunately, most of them are being conducted outside of the United States. A study in the Sudan compared two areas where the fluoride levels in the drinking water were 0.25 ppm in one area and 2.5 ppm in the other. Results showed no statistical difference in the dental decay rates between the two areas.

In Vancouver, which was never fluoridated, the cavity rate is lower than that of Toronto, which *is* fluoridated. A review of 214 selected water fluoridation studies published by the *British Medical Journal* in 2000, shows a tremendous lack of high quality research. The researchers note that the decay-reduction effects of fluoride have little scientific support and cite the studies they reviewed as poorly designed, with little regard for potentially contributing factors such as age, sex, ethnicity, tooth type (primary or permanent), use of fluoride, total fluoride consumption from all sources and method of measurement (clinical exam, photographic analysis, radiographs, etc.). In many of the studies that show fluoride to have an effect on tooth decay, the investigators fail to look at all the variables that could affect the outcome. And at the 1994 ADA Dietary Fluoride Supplement Conference, Brian A. Burt, MPH, Ph.D., a faculty member at the University of Michigan, argued that fluoride does not prevent dental decay in a manner significant enough to risk dental fluorosis and other health effects.

The CDC Study

When permanent molars erupt into a child's mouth, at age six and again at age 12, the grooves in the top of the teeth are not totally fused. This defect is a normal result of tooth development and these areas are usually the first to experience decay. In fact, 88% of tooth decay experienced by children is in the pit and fissures (grooves) of the back teeth. Since the early 1980s, quality dentists have put dental sealants in the grooves of these teeth to prevent decay from getting into the tooth and these have been a major success. Where children in their teenage years typically required six or eight dental fillings, the use of sealants means there is usually no decay present and no fillings required.

On 26 August 2005, the Center for Disease Control published its Morbidity and Mortality Weekly Reports (MMWR) Summary: *Surveillance for Dental Caries, Dental Sealants, Tooth Retention,*

Edentulism and Enamel Fluorosis, comparing statistics of decay among children and adults between 1988–1994 and 1999–2002. They arrived at four conclusions:

♦ There had been *no change* in the prevalence of dental decay in children's deciduous (baby) teeth between the two time periods.

♦ There had been *a reduction* in the prevalence of decay in permanent teeth of 10% for ages six to 19, and of 5+% for adults over 20 years of age. (See Graph 3-1.)

♦ There had been an *increase* of 13% in dental sealants among persons six to19. (See Graph 3-2.)

♦ A statistic about total tooth loss in the elderly (not relevant to this discussion).

People with a biased pro-fluoride opinion tend to conclude from this CDC study that fluoride was responsible for the reduction of decay in permanent teeth. Indeed, Graph 3-1 clearly shows a decrease of decay from a time with no fluoride use to a time with enormous fluoride use. The CDC's own final conclusions, however, rightly omit mentioning fluoride as the cause of the reduction. Though the authors *do* state that further surveillance tools are required to monitor fluoride exposure, they pointedly indicate that *fluoride had no effect on tooth decay*. The findings that the dental decay rates of two to 5-year-olds *increased* across the board, in spite of water fluoridation and ingested fluoride, are also noted by the Children's Dental Health Project.

The CDC authors, however, fail to consider that the study population—from 1988 to and through 2002—was the first in history to receive the dramatically increased application of dental sealants from the age of 6. Sealed permanent tooth surfaces increased 13% over the 14 years reviewed in this study. (See the Graph 3-2 showing increased sealant use.) Molars accounted for 85% of all sealed teeth. The fact that, in 2002, 32% of children and adolescents had sealed teeth is more than enough to explain any reduction in dental decay claimed for fluoride.

Prevalence of Dental Caries in Permanent Teeth★ Among Children and Adolescents Aged Six–19 Years, by Selected Characteristics

—United States, National Health and Nutrition Examination Survey. 1988–1994 and 1999–2002

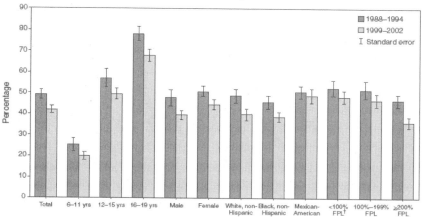

★Defined as having one or more decayed, missing, or filled surfaces in permanent tooth (DMFS>0) among those with at least one permanent tooth. All estimates are adjusted by age (single years) and sex to the US 2000 standard population, except sex, which is adjusted only by age.

† Percentage of the Federal Poverty Level (FPL). which varies by income and number of persons living in the household.

Graph 3-1: Decreased decay as reported in the CDC study

Dental Fluorosis—How Severe and How Common?

Dental fluorosis is the characteristic damage to tooth enamel associated with exposure to too much fluoride. We saw earlier how fluorosis was one of the early markers on the path that led to the elevation of fluoride as a cure-all for tooth decay.

The June 1994 issue of *Community Dental Oral Epidemiology* carried an article entitled "Trends in Prevalence of Dental Fluorosis in North America." It reported the prevalence of dental fluorosis ranged between 35% and 60% in water fluoridated communities and between 20% and 45% in non-fluoridated areas. Paul Connett, Ph.D., Professor of Chemistry at St. Lawrence University, Canton,

Prevalence of Dental Sealants in Children and Adolescents Aged Six–19 Years,* by Selected Characteristics

—United States, National Health and Nutrition Examination survey, 1988–1994 and 1999—2002

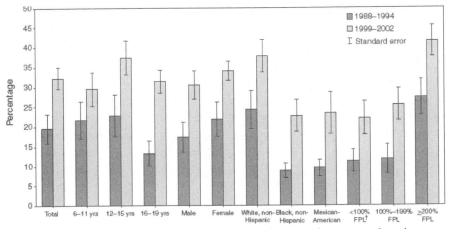

*Defined as having one or more permanent molar, premolar or upper lateral incisor with pit and fissure sealants. All estimates are adjusted by age (single years) and sex to the US 2000 population, except sex, which is adjusted only by age.
†Percentage of the Federal Poverty Level (FPL), which varies by income and number of persons living in the household.

Graph 3-2: Increased sealant use as reported in the CDC study

N.Y. cautioned, "If we couple this warning [fluoride damaged teeth] with an ever-growing body of peer-reviewed and published research which indicates fluoride's negative impact on the brain, the pineal gland (responsible for melatonin production) and the bone (osteosarcoma and hip fracture), our task is not to put more fluoride into the drinking water but to get it out." (See Figure 3-3, page 217.)

A review of scientific studies in Great Britain in 2000 indicated that 48% of children living in fluoridated communities had some degree of dental fluorosis. A study prepared by the WHO in 2000 and updated in 2005 compared tooth decay rates for 12-year-olds in fluoridated and non-fluoridated countries. Their data shows no statistical difference in decay rates between the two groups.

Since 1985, new studies have been published that support the longstanding contention of the US Natural Resources Defense Council and the US Environmental Protection Agency Union that moderate to severe dental fluorosis can indeed result in adverse health effects. The US Environmental Protection Agency itself has steadfastly refused to entertain the concept that dental fluorosis is a sign of general fluoride toxicity in the whole body. For over 30 years they have called this condition a "cosmetic aberration" and refused to consider scientific data from reputable sources in the scientific and toxicological communities. The EPA claims that if there was evidence of serious health effects, they would lower the MCLG from the current 4 ppm to below 2 ppm. In all probability they would not remove fluoride totally from additives given the pressure from the ADA and others who refuse to examine this data.

Three general categories of research now appear, any of which should have been sufficient to define dental fluorosis as an adverse health effect that should require authorities to lower the maximum contaminant level goal (MCLG) to less than 2 ppm.

Fluorosis/Psychological Effects

In 1984 the US National Institute of Mental Health advised the EPA that moderate or severe fluorosis would adversely affect a child's psychological development because of the embarrassment of chronically brown, black and pitted teeth. The EPA responded that there was no scientific basis for that claim.

A study conducted in April of 2006 at the Wales College of Medicine, UK, concluded that "attribution of characteristics that go beyond the aesthetic are significantly influenced by altered tooth appearances." Participants in this study viewed images of dental fluorosis and dental decay and were asked to give opinions. The images of severe fluorosis had a significant negative impact on social judgments. The afflicted were judged less intelligent, less reliable, less hygienic, less social and less attractive. Worse still, obvious untreated dental decay rated even lower on a scale of social acceptability.

Fluorosis/Cavities

It would seem elementary to anyone who has seen many cases of dental fluorosis that such damaged tooth structure would make the tooth more susceptible to decay. However the EPA recorded no studies that reached that conclusion. There are however at least eight studies since 1985 indicating increased tooth decay associated with fluorosis. Two of these studies from 2003 [cited by the US Agency of Toxic Substance and Disease Registry (ATSDR)], concluded that dental fluorosis increases the incidence of caries, erosion and tooth fracture. According to the US ATSDR, "in more severely fluorosed teeth, the enamel is pitted and discolored and is prone to fracture and wear."

Fluorosis/Bone Fractures

Many committees and researchers have noted that adverse disruption of normal mineralization of developing teeth would probably indicate a parallel disruption in mineralization of osseous structures. Some have recommended to the EPA that research be done to assess the relationship between dental fluorosis and bone development. No significant research has been published in the United States in the last 20 years but studies have been conducted outside the US. In the next section, we'll look closely at these wider effects.

FLUORIDE TOXICITY: THE WHOLE BODY

If fluoride's only effects were those on the teeth, well, most responsible researchers would still warn against its use. But the tragic fact is that fluoride damage to teeth is just the beginning—a toxic warning sign. In this section, we're going to look at this toxin's real potential.

General Fluorosis

Fluoride can attack almost every system in the human body. The effects of chronic exposure are neither acute nor instantaneous and hence damage can accumulate in the tissues before it is recognized. It's always difficult for scientists and doctors (and public health officials) to detect damage caused by slow progressive degenerative disorders because the effects mimic many others medical conditions. In this respect fluoride poisoning is similar to mercury overexposure; they both manifest health conditions that are not readily attributable to the exposure. Simply look at lead poisoning: it took decades for the medical community to make the connection between exposure and ingestion of lead and the decrease in cognitive abilities and IQ that is its

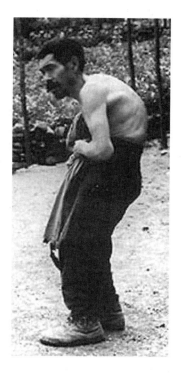

Figure 3-4: A Mexican man showing the effects of fluorosis.

consequence. How long had asbestos been used until the connection was made between exposure to asbestos and lung disease or cancer development?

A.K. Susheela, an epidemiologist and expert on hydrofluorosis in India, has extensively studied the extreme effects of this disease. In India there are an estimated 62 million people suffering from fluorosis—the disease. Most of cases are the result of naturally occurring excess fluoride in local drinking water. According to the World Health Organization guidelines, the maximum permissible limit is 1 mg of fluoride per liter. Those regions of India severely affected demonstrate levels in the 5 to 23 mg per liter concentration. The

Public Health Engineering Department (PHE) found that in the villages in these regions, nearly one in four persons were found to have a fluoride-related disease.

There is much overlap of degenerative fluoride-exposure conditions. We're going to look quickly at the effects on separate body systems, but the total effects are always multiple.

Toxic Cellular Effects

The disruptive effects of fluoride at a cellular level have not been widely investigated. One study has shown that sodium fluoride alters the RHO

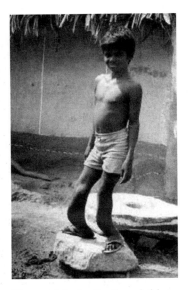

Figure 3-5: An Indian child, a victim of fluorosis

pathway (responsible for actin organization, gene expression and cell cycle progression) of cellular differentiation of ameloblasts and causes alterations in the actin cytoskeleton. The bottom line is that this can lead to alterations in genetic expression.

Serious developmental consequences can result because changes at a cellular level might affect the "blueprints" that form other tissues. Recent studies have shown that

♦ Excess fluoride can cause normal "programmed" cell death (normal aging) to occur abnormally earlier in animal models.

♦ Fluoride can cause changes in cell reproduction in our bodies in both oral tissues and the liver (animal models).

♦ When human embryo liver cells were challenged with fluoride, lipid peroxidation (a toxic result of fatty metabolism) and DNA damage were observed.

♦ When liver cells adversely affected by fluoride were exposed to selenium, partial protection was afforded by the selenium against the fluoride damage.

♦ In an animal model, exposure to fluoride limits the ability of the body to appropriately dispose of toxic substances. This causes accumulation of other reactive substances (e.g. free radicals and compounds that can cause tissue damage) with adverse health effects.

Skeletal Fluorosis

I've mentioned Dr. Hardy Limeback earlier in the book. Dr. Limeback is a dentist who heads the Department of Preventive Dentistry at the University of Toronto and is past-president of the Canadian Association for Dental Research. He has conducted studies of residents of Toronto, which has been fluoridated since 1964.

"Fluoride's adverse effects occur upon ingestion," he reports. "Fluoride gets into every cell of the body and can especially damage the bones and teeth." He states that *half of all fluoride stays in the skeletal system and accumulates with age.* His data shows that Toronto residents have twice the amount of fluoride in their hip bones as residents of non-fluoridated Montreal. And from his research he makes this worrying observation: "We discovered that fluoride is actually altering the basic architecture of human bones."

Meanwhile, there's an increasing incidence of osteoporosis and osteopenia among Americans, and in people of younger and younger ages. Drugs such as Fossomax™ are marketed as able to help the body retain calcium instead of metabolizing and excreting it. But all the drugs available cannot help if there is an underlying physical change taking place in the basic architecture of the bones, a change that is causing an increase in bone brittleness. This appears to be what is happening with the long-term ingestion of fluoride. And if that isn't bad enough, fluoride is now known to be toxic to bone, actually causing its destruction.

A 2001 study in Mexico assessed the incidence of bone fractures among children and adults living in a high-fluoride area of the country. Although fluoride concentrations in the public drinking water in Mexico are regulated to below 1.5%, endemic fluorosis is a problem in regions of naturally occurring high fluoride content. This study was conducted in one of those areas, where the drinking-water fluoride levels are in the 1.54 to 5.67 ppm range (not too much higher than public fluoridated water levels in the USA). Results showed that the *higher the fluoride levels in the drinking water, the higher the risk of dental fluorosis and the higher the incidence of bone fractures.* Conversely, the higher the occurrence of fractures, the higher the fluoride levels detected (Graph 3-3).

> ...the higher the fluoride levels in the drinking water, the higher the risk of dental fluorosis and the higher the incidence of bone fractures.

In a US study published in the *British Medical Journal* in October. 2000, Dr. Kathy Phipps reported older white women living in fluoridated water communities for over 20 years to have a 32% higher rate of wrist fractures than women living in other communities. The overall bone density of several other osseous areas showed no significant changes. The study made no effort to determine any mineral or fluoride consumption over the same period that would have impacted the results.

In the past 15 years, four studies have been published in the *Journal of the American Medical Association* that link the ingestion of fluoridated tap water to an increased risk of hip fracture.

Even the initial Newburgh-Kingston Study, its organizers busy touting the benefits of fluoridation, revealed adverse health effects from the fluoride ingestion. Knee x-rays taken of Newburgh children reveal cortical bone defects and irregular mineralization of the thigh bone. These safety studies were never publicly revealed.

Many studies, such as ones conducted in Toronto, in Scandinavia and in Rochester, Minnesota, demonstrate that, although individuals exposed to fluoride show an increase in the mass and height of

Bone Fractures vs Dean Dental Fluorosis Index

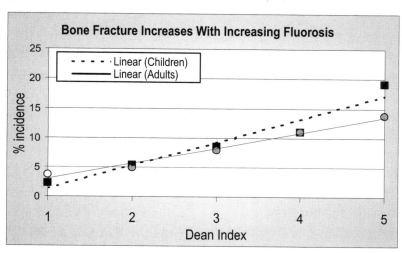

SOURCE: Alarcon-Herrera IMIT, et al. (2001). Well Water Fluoride, Dental fluorosis. Bone Fractures in the Guadiana Valley of Mexico. Fluoride 34(2):139-149.

Graph 3-3: Incidence of bone fractures increase with increasing fluoride intake

the trabecular component of bone (the inside bone structure), there is *no* correlation with an increase in bone strength. Instead, actual bone quality is poor and there appears to be an increase in bone fractures and an increase in immobilizing conditions. The changes in bone composition show an actual loss of trabecular strength with over- or under-mineralized bone. In the *Journal of the American Medical Association* in 1992, Danielson found that the risk of hip fracture was approximately 30% higher for women and 40% higher for men exposed to fluoridated (1 ppm) drinking water when compared to those drinking nonfluoridated water. The fluoride-induced changes cause an increase of the bone mass inside the bones, but a decrease in strength of the outside cortical bone surface. The result can be a three-fold increase in bone fractures compared to non-fluoride subjects.

Other studies in Finland demonstrate that the longer people drink fluoridated water and the higher the concentration of the fluoride, the more fluoride accumulates in the bone structure. This has been associated with increases in osteoporosis, osteomalacia and osteofluorosis, all capable of increasing brittle bone disease.

Long-term fluoride ingestion (over six years) causes changes in how bone is structured, causing it to be more brittle and prone to fracture. These effects are worse where fluoride exposure occurs before menopause in women.

Some studies do not take into account the pathogenesis of osseous changes with long-term fluoride exposure. Simply reporting study results is not enough. A 1980 study in Finland, for example, attempted to show no difference in bone mineral density between fluoridated and non-fluoridated areas. However they failed to examine factors other than cancellous bone content (the type of bone structure inside the hard outer type in long bones) when measuring strength. The discussion and conclusions of studies must include not just the fluoride exposure but all influencing factors—called confounding factors—that could affect the bone changes. These other biological influences must be included if we're to understand the significance of the long-term fluoride findings.

> In the *Journal of the American Medical Association* in 1992, Danielson found that the risk of hip fracture was approximately 30% higher for women and 40% higher for men exposed to fluoridated (1 ppm) drinking water when compared to those drinking nonfluoridated water.

♦ Bone is rapidly being reformed and changed prior to menopause in women. After menopause, much less osseous turnover occurs. Consequently if fluoride is involved post menopause, the results will be radically different than if fluoride exposure occurs earlier in life for several years.

♦ Increase bone mass does *not* mean stronger bone resistance to fracture. Calcium conservation in bone is more a result of hormonal production and activity than dietary calcium intake. Proges-terone and testosterone stimu-late increased bone formation, while estrogen decreases bone loss. Diet, exercise, exposure to xenobiotics (pesticides of all sorts), and genetic factors all af-fect sex hormone production.

> Long-term fluoride ingestion (over six years) causes changes in how bone is structured, causing it to be more brittle and prone to fracture. These effects are worse where fluo-ride exposure occurs before menopause in women.

Oh No! Another!

It may seem scarcely credible that I have to reveal yet another scandal in the course of the fluoride story. This is an ugly one and may be especially disturbing for Cana-dians, who still revere the memory of Terry Fox, the young man who died of cancer while running across the continent to bring at-tention to the disease that cost him his leg and ultimately his life.

In 1977 the US National Academy of Sciences (NAS) reviewed the safety record of fluoride in drinking water. The results revealed a 13.5% incidence in bone structure defects in the population of Newburgh, NY, as we know, the site of the nation's first experi-ment in fluoridated drinking water, fluoridated since the 1950s. By contrast, the incidence of these defects in Kingston, NY, the com-munity in the study which has never been fluoridated, was only 7%. The NAS at that time recommended a study to assess the potential for osteosarcoma (bone cancer) in young boys from fluoride inges-tion. The resulting study by the US Public Health Service (USPHS) was completed in 1991 and showed a significant association between fluoride exposure and osteosarcoma in boys. This study by the Na-tional Cancer Institute (taken from records 1973 through 1987) showed a 79% *increase* in bone cancer in fluoridated communities during that time, compared to 4% *decrease* for non-fluoridated communities. When expanded nationwide the disparity between fluoridated and non-fluoridated communities held.[2]

The Environmental Working Group (EWG) of Washington, DC has pursued this information and petitioned the National Institutes of Environmental Health Sciences (NIEHS) to investigate a cover-up of relevant scientific studies demonstrating the potential of fluoride to cause cancer in boys. The NIEHS had issued a grant to the Harvard University School of Dental Medicine in 2001 under the auspices of Dr. Chester Douglass, chairman of the Department of Oral Health Policy and Epidemiology. The doctoral dissertation by Elise B. Bassin was titled "Age-specific Fluoride Exposure in Drinking Water and Osteosarcoma (United States)." Her conclusions

> ...verified the association between fluoride exposure in drinking water during childhood and the incidence of osteosarcoma among males.

It's to be expected that this investigation would have set off fireworks of concern over fluoride exposure. Instead Dr. Douglass submitted a report, as advisor for Dr. Bassin, to the NIEHS with conclusions totally contradicting the results of her thesis. Dr. Douglass cited only two references, the Bassin reference being one, but neglected to note her conclusions. He concluded there was *no evidence* of an association between fluoride and osteosarcoma.

Such a serious misrepresentation of unbiased research results by Dr. Douglass appears to be in direct violation of federal research guidelines. One might expect Dr. Douglass to have been prosecuted for federal violations—or censored at least by the Harvard School of Dental Medicine. And indeed, in a closed-door hearing by the

---

[2] See www.ewg.org, letters to NIEHS dated June 27, 2005, to the National Toxicology Program dated June 6, 2005 and to Dr. Chester Douglas dated June 23, 2005

Harvard Ethics Panel, Dr. Chester Douglass' flagrant violation of evidence was reviewed and Dr. Douglass was found *not responsible* for any omissions or errors in the federal grant. And in September 2006, Dr. Chester Douglass made a one million dollar contribution to the University's Dental School. And as it turns out—oh Reader, steel yourself—Dr. Chester Douglass was an employee of the Colgate toothpaste company and had heartily advocated fluoride in Colgate's journal "The Oral Care Report."

In October 2006, the Environmental Working Group sent a letter of protest to the president of Harvard University to express their members' joint displeasure at the way Dr. Douglass' hearing had been held in secret and no transcripts released. They called for a complete disclosure. They're still waiting. If this could happen at a respected school such as Harvard, can there be any doubt that ordinary doctors can sometimes have hidden reasons for their actions?

Cardiac Effects

Investigators at the Suleyman Demirel University Medical School in Turkey, have demonstrated in animal studies that long-term exposure (defined as more than six months) to sodium fluoride in drinking water changes the composition of myocardial tissue. Higher intake of fluoride resulted in myocardial cell damage and necrosis (death of heart muscle cells) and alteration of the normal anatomy of the heart muscle tissues.

Gastrointestinal Effects

If you were to swallow a 1 mg fluoride tablet or drink fluoridated water containing 1 mg of fluoride, you could expect to experience acute fluoride poisoning. The effects appear to arise from fluoride's direct contact with the lining of the stomach. Severe vomiting, nausea and abdominal pain are the most common symptoms. The American Association of Poison Control Centers reports 10% of children who ingested 5 to 9 mg of fluoride experienced vomiting. In 1990, researchers at a school of dentistry in Sweden reported that dental topical fluoride treatments with fluoride gels (1.23% fluoride) caused 40% of the applied fluoride to be retained in the stomach. Damage to mucosal stomach tissues, including erosions of the lining of the stomach, was observed in 70% of the subjects. A full 90% of the subjects showed cellular disruptions of the stomach lining.

In cases of gastrointestinal symptoms arising from chronic fluoride exposure, discontinuance of the fluoride resulted in reduction or elimination of the symptoms.

Non-ulcer dyspepsia—we know it as indigestion—can be caused by fluoride toxicity. The ingested fluoride is transformed in the stomach into hydrofluoric acid, which corrodes the epithelial lining of the gastrointestinal tract and, not surprisingly, causes pain.

> Higher intake of fluoride resulted in myocardial cell damage and necrosis (death of heart muscle cells) and alteration of the normal anatomy of the heart muscle tissues.

Reproductive Effects

Since fluoride was first introduced to public water supplies, studies have been published that demonstrate the toxic effects of fluoride exposure to the human reproductive system. Studies based on the fluoridated city of Newburgh, where the claims of fluoride dental benefits were born in 1956, showed girls to begin their menarche (onset of menstruation) almost six months earlier, on average, than those living in Kingston, NY, a non-fluoridated city. These findings were never publicly reported, though this early "maturation" effect was confirmed in an animal study by Jennifer Luke, in 1997, at the School of Biological Sciences in the United Kingdom.

Dr. Luke investigated the early onset of puberty again in 2001.

Her research relates this change in physiology to fluoride accumulation in the pineal gland, located at the base of the brain and responsible for the synthesis and metabolism of serotonin and melatonin. The fluoride was found to inhibit synthesis of melatonin and thereby trigger the early puberty. Conversely male sexual maturation was stunted and the mean testes weight of males exposed to fluoride was significantly lower. The pineal gland and melatonin synthesis is intimately involved with many regulatory systems in the body, especially its role in aging and cancer.

In 1991 the US Department of Health and Human Services, in their "Review of Fluoride: Benefits and Risks," recommended additional study to investigate the relationship between fluoride and the reproductive system.

Several human epidemiological studies draw a correlation between decreasing total fertility rate (TFR) and increasing fluoride levels in the body. Countries with lower fertility rates had 3 ppm (only 3 ppm!) fluoride in their water supply. The researchers suspect that lower levels of circulating testosterone and observable toxic effects on Sertoli cells and gonadotrophs contribute to the reduced TFR. Lowered birth rates were observed in most groups subjected to increased fluoride levels, again as low as 3 ppm.

Neurological Effects

Dr. Phyllis Mullenix of the at Forsyth Dental Center in Boston, Massachusetts, was the head of the first dental toxicology department in any research facility in the world. Her expertise was the detection of neurotoxicity and her first studies on fluoride neurotoxicity were undertaken in 1987. The results of her research were published in 1995. Her initial research findings, supported by subsequent research studies, showed unique and unexpected results. Animal studies demonstrated early exposure to fluoride resulted in *changes in brain function*. This result was seen as significant because the fluoride plasma levels in the animals (0.059 to 0.640 ppm) were similar to those reported in humans exposed to similar levels of fluoride. The effects were age specific: adults exposed to fluoride showed cognitive deficits (decreased mental acuity, lowered IQ and impairment of memory), while prenatal exposure to fluoride (if a mother was living in a fluoridated drinking water community for instance) exhibited hyperactivity behavior as well. Specific areas of the brain, especially the hippocampus, showed an affinity for fluoride accumulation. The higher the level of fluoride exposure, the more accumulation of fluoride in the brain. There was real potential for motor dysfunction, IQ deficits and learning disabilities. Two studies in China show an average decrease in IQ of 10 points in 8- to thirteen-year-olds drinking fluoridated water over the course of their young lives.

Mullenix's team discovered that, at high levels of fluoride in drinking water (3 to 11 ppm), the osseous deformities were bypassed and the central nervous system was directly affected. The usual skeletal changes from a toxic fluoride exposure were *not* there to alert the clinicians of possible brain dysfunction.

> The higher the level of fluoride exposure, the more accumulation of fluoride in the brain. There was real potential for motor dysfunction, IQ deficits and learning disabilities.

One of her major concerns was that these toxic children could have as much as *10 times* the maximum plasma levels of fluoride only one hour after they received a topical fluoride gel treatment in a dental office. The children were being exposed to levels of fluoride that were known to alter their behavior. Symptoms of long-term fluoride overexposure in adults were impaired memory and concentration, and lethargy, headache, depression and confusion.

Other studies reveal that chronic exposure to fluoride as low as 1 ppm both compromises the blood brain barrier and *increases aluminum concentrations* in brain tissues. Varner suggests additional research is needed to reveal the role fluoride plays in neurodegenerative diseases. Other studies in China and India, where endemic excessive fluoride levels exist naturally in the drinking water, have indicated that ingesting high levels of fluoride can also lead to *hearing* impairment and cretinism.

Hematological Effects

E. Eren, from the Department of Pediatrics of the Suleyman Demirel University Medical School in Turkey, conducted an animal study in 1995 in a region of Turkey where fluorosis is endemic. Administration of excess fluoride caused more than a ⅓ reduction in white blood cell count. Additional abnormal developmental changes were observed in granulocytes in the bone marrow.

Thyroid Effects

Disturbances in human thyroid function have far-reaching effects on regulatory mechanisms and the development of body systems far beyond simple iodine metabolism. It has been well documented that fluoride interferes with enzymes produced in the thyroid gland. These iodothyronine deiodinases act as catalysts in the metabolism of iodine. This enzyme activity is necessary for proper thyroid function. Symptoms of hypothyroidism, which is especially prevalent in women 40 years of age and

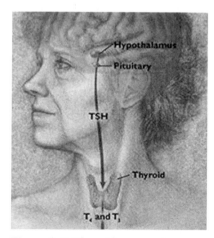

Figure 3-7: Thyroid connections (courtesy www.fluoridealert.org).

older, are fatigue, depression, weight gain, hair loss, muscle pains, increased levels of "bad" cholesterol (LDL), and heart disease. Synthroid is the number five prescribed drug in the United States and is used to treat hypothyroidism.

In New Delhi, India, a 2005 study of children who were exposed to various levels of fluoride in drinking water, showed fluoride levels in their blood and urine above current *upper* limits. These findings held even in the *control groups* that the ADA and EPA would consider as ingesting "safe levels of fluoride." Subclinical hypothyroidism was diagnosed in roughly half of the sample group, but also in 19% of the control group. The study showed that fluoride in excess may be inducing disease normally attributed to iodine deficiency. Fluoride and iodide are in some respects related halogens. The physical degenerative changes to children affected in this manner are permanent.

We know that fluoride is lethal to the thyroid gland because, until about 1970, fluoride (in doses as low as 2 mg/day or as high as 10 mg/day) was used as an anti-thyroid drug for patients with hyperthyroidism. Many people living in fluoridated communities are ingesting 1.6 to 6.6 mg of fluoride a day, within old treatment levels that attacked thyroid function.

The largest US study ever conducted on maternal iodine deficiency—by the Foundation for Blood Research, Scarborough, Maine, published in 1999—showed that even mild (not readily observable) subclinical hypothyroidism in the mother resulted in lowered IQ in the child.

Clinical Manifestations of General Fluorosis

The truly astonishing effects of chronic fluoride exposure have emerged from regions where high natural fluoride levels have caused serious health effects to the local populations. Efforts to eliminate this fluoride scourge by remedial measures directed at the source of fluoride appears to lead to complete relief of many of the earliest toxic symptoms, some resolving within two weeks. But tragically, the majority of serious physical and metabolic aberrations from fluoride poisoning are permanent.

Long-term exposure to fluoride can occur naturally in communities where fluoride levels in the drinking water are excessively high. Studies conducted in those rural areas of Mexico, India and China where the only source of water is from a community well have revealed some of the health changes—often present as more routine diseases—that result from this overexposure. The following may impress you with the insidious nature of this chemical attack.

As I previously noted, where fluorosis is not too advanced, there is hope of reversing some of its effects. The two interventions necessary to achieve this goal are:

> If your child has symptoms of hypothyroidism, even if iodine supplementation is being prescribed, his or her fluoride levels must be tested! Fluoride is lethal to the thyroid gland.

1. Removal of all sources of ingested fluoride, including drinking water, foods and beverages that may contain fluoride, to achieve zero ingestion (or a maximum exposure of less than 1 ppm total).
2. Nutritional supplementation with Vitamins C and E, calcium and antioxidants.

During the one-year follow-up that was part of the fluorosis study in India, researchers found these measures to have helped the stricken population.

Signs and Symptoms of General Fluorosis

This list of basic signs and symptoms is by no means complete. As with most toxic materials (such as mercury in dental fillings), the effects may not be direct or immediately visible.

♦ Aches and pains in the joints without visible signs of fluid accumulation, arthritis. Body pain, joint arthritic (knee) pain and (lower) back pain.

♦ Painful, restricted movement, stiff joints

♦ Non-ulcer dyspepsia (acid stomach or indigestion) with nausea, pain in the stomach, bloated or gas sensation, constipation followed by diarrhea (irritable bowel). Affects similar to irritable bowel syndrome (IBS).

♦ Frequent urination (polyuria) and excessive thirst (polydypsia).

♦ Nervousness, depression and paresthesia or tingling in the fingers and toes.

♦ Muscle weakness, fatigue (loss of energy) and anemia with low hemoglobin level.

♦ Repeated abortion/still births.

♦ Full-term, low birthweight babies

♦ Male infertility with abnormal sperm morphology, low testosterone levels, abnormal sperm counts.

Diagnosis

Investigators can determine the seriousness of suspected fluorosis using three initial tests:

♦ They measure the fluoride levels in drinking water, urine and blood (serum). A 24-hour urine collection is preferred. Samples are collected in plastic bottles, not glass, which contains silica that can react with fluoride.

♦ They take x-rays of the area where the pain and stiffness is located.

♦ They x-ray the forearm to look for interosseous membrane calcification. Fluoride damage causes calcification of the joint ligaments and in the forearm, this damage does not mimic other orthopedic conditions.

THE WORLD OF DENTAL FLUORIDE

We've devoted the past section to the toxic effects of fluoride, whether it occurs naturally in drinking water or is introduced deliberately, effects that have ranged from the cosmetically deleterious to the tragically destructive.

Now I must turn to what my profession—dentistry—has seen fit to do with fluoride.

How and Why

Since the 1950s, in the wake of our story, fluoride has been promoted by dentists and toothpaste manufacturers as the primary method of preventing tooth decay and to a lesser extent making teeth less sensitive. Dentists are in no hurry to change this approach.

Dentistry and medicine are similar in that practices should constantly change as new materials are developed and new diagnostic and treatment methods emerge. But as we've seen, not all dentists keep up with current research concerning materials and procedures that they use every day in their offices. There are, of course, periodicals and services that review the immense volume of published literature and clinical studies to summarize them for the clinician. Yet many practitioners continue to ignore these advances and practice outdated dentistry.

Here's an example. For decades, dentists drilled out decay and old fillings with a drill (called a "handpiece") that was slow compared to those used today. The drilling bur revolved at 5,000 to 20,0000 revolutions per minute. Tooth structure is exceptionally hard and it would take a while to sufficiently drill into the tooth to create a proper hole for a filling to be placed. To make matters worse there was no anesthesia given for routine fillings. The patient could actually smell the tooth heating up and almost burning! Then, in the 1950s, high-speed water-cooled handpieces were produced and made available to dentists. These were light years ahead of what they had been using. The drilling bur rotated at 3 to 4,000,000 revolutions per minute and could prepare a cavity for a filling in minutes.

It may surprise you to learn that it was years before most dentists switched over to these new drills. Why? Because, as we know, it's intimidating and scary when you have to make major changes in how you do things, things that seemed so comfortable for years. Dentists had not received training in this new equipment at dental school and were unsure how to effectively use it.

So before we can look at how most dentists use fluoride in their practices, let's look at *how* dentists make decisions to change the procedures and techniques they use to treat patients.

The Current Standard of Care

"Standard of care" is a medical/dental/legal term. It means different things to each professional group. The professional organizations for general dentistry and the dental specialties each have committees that set down basic patient-care procedures, the "minimum level of care" or the "parameters of care" that they believe should be followed by all practitioners during diagnosis and treatment. Most of these basic procedures or guidelines are published and available to the members of the organizations. In dentistry, one set of "standards of care" is established by the American Dental Association, another by the US Academy of General Dentistry for general dentists. These standards are generally rooted in what is now called "evidence-based dentistry," the evidence being the scientific studies and clinical trials published in journals, newsletters, websites and elsewhere. The associations try to present a fair and balanced argument for practicing a certain way and offer clinicians their rationale for preferentially using certain procedures. The actual written standards are so basic that it is hard for any practitioner to knowingly violate them.[3]

Now comes the catch. For a scientific study or clinical-trial result to be published, the author of the study must present material that the editorial staff of the journal and the "peer reviewers"—

well-established and respected clinicians who agree to review articles submitted to a journal—will approve. It's common knowledge that many professional journals tend to publish only certain well-connected clinicians' studies, or studies from high-profile universities, while ignoring other studies from "outside" authors. A little-known clinician has small chance of getting a controversial treatment study (that is, one whose findings run contrary to established opinion) published in a major journal such as *Lancet, New England Journal of Medicine* or the *Journal of the American Dental Association*. If the editorial staff or peer reviewers do *not* agree with the interpretation of a study's results, either group may block the publishing of the study. Sure, the blocking of a single study isn't going to much affect the daily practice of medicine or dentistry. But the blocking of several studies that point in a certain direction may represent a bias—a "prescreening"—in a journal that clinicians rely on for evidence—and may indeed have an effect on practice. If selected results of selected studies are used to support accepted ideas, the journal may be in effect denying clinicians the opportunity to review and consider new evidence for themselves, evidence that they could use to make their own decisions as how to best practice medicine or dentistry.

The suggestion that national associations are subtly controlling how clinicians'—including dentists'—practices may sound like paranoia, but the subtle influence of a journal's editorial staff and peer reviewers, an influence that determines what readers will and will not be allowed to read, is an established step in the publication of

[3] ACCME Content Validation Statement
Accredited providers are responsible for validating the clinical content of CME [continuing medical education] activities that they provide. Specifically,
1. All the recommendations involving clinical medicine in a CME activity must be based on evidence that is accepted within the profession of medicine as adequate justification for their indications and contraindications in the care of patients.
2. All scientific research referred to, reported or used in CME in support or justification of a patient care recommendation must conform to the generally accepted standards of experimental design, data collection and analysis.

scientific study and clinica-trial results. This bias is not obvious to clinicians or to their patients.

In my opinion, it is the responsibility of every clinician to investigate for themselves the pros and cons of diagnoses and procedures supported by any specific journal or organization. I would never have understood the dangers of fluoride and mercury in the dental office without reading scientific studies and clinical trials published in journals other than those published by—and approved by—the various conventional dental associations.

Here's another instance of bias. The American Dental Association has published letters and articles galore illustrating how fluoride has safely reduced decay levels. They have rarely published any of the scientific findings showing the permanent damage fluoride does to adult teeth in children or the bone changes that take place in younger and older adults exposed to fluoride over long periods of time, as in the case of fluoridated water. Yet the damage caused by fluoride exposure is a fact, as we've seen.

With this "filter" in mind, this "control" that can be the medical publishing industry, let's turn now to the various applications of fluoride that dentists are supposed to recommend.

Topical Fluoride Treatment for Children: Just Open Up and Say No

The vast majority of dental offices in the United States recommend the application of fluoride to children's teeth following the cleaning and polishing that is part of a regular dental checkup. This amounts to a treatment every six months. In most American states, the procedure must by law be performed only by a dentist or dental hygienist. The ADA recommends topical fluoride treatments for children of six months to 16 years of age. Placing their faith in 50-year-old studies supported by the US Public Health Department and American Dental Association, most dentists believe the following:

♦ Fluoride topically applied to the tooth surface inhibits tooth decay.

♦ Fluoride topically applied is somehow absorbed into the tooth surface itself.

♦ Fluoride treatments keep working against decay long after the actual application to the teeth.

♦ Fluoride has no systemic effects on whole-body systems.

Unfortunately scientific and medical research does not support any of these points except the first statement, and that only in part. I'm going to show you incontrovertible evidence that the sole decay-preventive effect from fluoride occurs briefly and only while the fluoride is present in the mouth. Worse, fluoride does far more long-term damage to whole-body systems than previously suspected.

But I'm running ahead here. For now, let's look closely at the technique dentists are taught for the application of topical fluoride.

Empty fluoride trays are tried in the child's mouth to confirm the tray size is correct. Two trays are used per treatment, one for the upper or maxillary arch and one for the lower or mandibular arch. The fluoride medium is supplied to the dentist as a gel, foam or solution. There are several types of fluoride chemicals of several concentrations. The trays have a trough or U-shape all the way around to hold the fluoride-containing material until the tray is inserted in the child's mouth. When inserted onto the arch being treated, the fluoride material squishes up around the teeth for the prescribed period of time, usually three or four minutes. Excess fluoride invariably leaks and flows out of the tray. The child is told to try not to swallow the fluoride "stuff" while the trays are in their mouth. Although the child has a saliva ejector tube hanging in the bottom of the mouth to suck out excess fluids while the dentist or dental hygienist is working, the child naturally swallows some fluoride. Children can't help it. At the end of the prescribed time, the trays are removed and the child is told to spit out any excess liquid into the sink. The child and parent are instructed to refrain from any food or beverage for a period of time to allow the fluoride to stay on the surface of the teeth—usually one-half to one hour after the treatment.

Most topical fluoride treatments are given to children right through the early teenage years. Occasionally one of my adult patients who believed the hype about fluoride's anti-cavity action would specifically request a treatment immediately following their scaling and polishing by my hygienist. However this happened infrequently, probably because dental insurance companies do not cover adult fluoride treatments.

> Dental students are taught that excess fluoride swallowed by a child may cause seizures, coma or death.

The techniques and rational for topical fluoride treatments are taught in dental school. Students learn that fluoride is toxic if ingested in larger than "therapeutic amounts." They learn to recommend and administer topical fluoride treatments for children to strengthen erupting teeth against decay, but they're never taught how fluoride interacts with the tooth surface to make teeth stronger or offered any scientific proof that it does. The safety and efficacy of topical fluoride is an article of faith.

But consider this: dental students are cautioned *not* to administer fluoride treatments to children who are "too young." These patients may not understand the critical instructions or cooperate with the safety regime. After the trays are removed, the little tykes may actually swallow excess fluoride instead of properly expectorating. Dental students are taught that excess fluoride swallowed by a child may cause seizures, coma or death. Should the child swallow too much fluoride during the procedure, the dentist is supposed to insure the child *immediately* drinks milk or antacids in a liquid or gel formulation. The calcium in these products binds the excess fluoride in the stomach and prevents it from being absorbed by the gastrointestinal system. As we'll see, calcium and fluoride bind so tightly within the cellular structure of the body, the calcium cannot be available for bone growth, muscle function and nerve conduction.

But the dentist cannot see or measure the amount of fluoride in the trays anyway. So how is she supposed to know how much fluoride the child has ingested?

Parent must ask themselves, then, how well can this archaic and grossly dangerous technique work to prevent cavities safely if:

Dental insurance companies do not cover adult fluoride treatments. Do they know something the public doesn't know?

♦ It is so toxic it can lead to death?

♦ The dentist cannot tell if the child is overdosing on the fluoride?

♦ The child cannot eat or drink because it will remove the fluoride and leave no protection on the tooth?

♦ The fluoride binds calcium so strongly it prevents calcium from being used for other needs of the body?

Oral Fluoride Supplementation for Children

The US Center for Disease Control, the CDC, in its fluoride document, a part of the 2001 Morbidity and Mortality Weekly Report (MMWR), recommends doctors prescribe dietary fluoride supplements according to the dosage schedule shown in Table 1.

They caution against doctors prescribing any of these supplements until they have conducted a complete evaluation of any pros and cons that may arise from an assessment of the patient's health. Although this includes an analysis of the fluoride levels in the patient's drinking water, *no mention* is made about the risks of high fluoride intake such as those provided in supplements, or of the whole-body health effects of overexposure. The only caution noted by the CDC about excessive fluoride is the appearance of enamel fluorosis, which is noted as a cosmetic aberration affecting developing teeth. Yet current toxicology expert opinion considers the appearance of fluorotic teeth as the *earliest sign of fluoride overdosage*.

The American Dental Association has changed its rules and regulations concerning fluoride so many times, it's difficult for dentists to decide when and if and at what level fluoride supplements should be prescribed. With the advisory to evaluate the patient's current exposure to other sources of fluoride, the ADA has made it almost impossible for a dentist to efficiently evaluate if their child-patient should get additional supplementation. How can a dentist readily determine the fluoride in the water the patient drinks? Water where? At home? At school? At the gym? At a friend's house? How can a dentist know what foods a child-patient may eat? Where? How was it prepared? How much toothpaste does the child swallow? In 1994 the ADA rewrote the Fluoride Supplement Dosage Schedule so that it takes into account the local fluoridated water in the community in which the patient lives. They caution the doctor to evaluate the *total fluoride intake of the patient before prescribing any*

TABLE 1. Recommended dietary fluoride supplement* schedule

Age	Fluoride concentration in community drinking water[1]		
	<0.3 ppm	0.3–0.6 ppm	>0.6 ppm
0–6 months	None	None	None
6 months–3 years	0.25 mg/day	None	None
3–6 years	0.50 mg/day	0.25 mg/day	None
6–16 years	1.0 mg/day	0.50 mg/day	None

* Sodium fluoride (2.2 mg sodium fluoride contains 1 mg fluoride ion).
[1] 1.0 parts per million (ppm) = 1 mg/L.
Sources:
Meskin LH, ed. Caries diagnosis and risk assessment: a review of preventive strategies and management. J Am Dent Assoc 1995;126(suppl):1S–24S.
American Academy of Pediatric Dentistry. Special issue: reference manual 1994–95. Pediatr Dent 1995;16(special issue):1–96.
American Academy of Pediatrics Committee on Nutrition. Fluoride supplementation for children: interim policy recommendations. Pediatrics 1995;95:777.

Table 3-2: The CDC's fluoride recommendations

fluoride supplements. Of course that's effectively impossible. There's an abundance of fluoride in foods and drinks.

So the ADA now recommends the use of daily dietary fluoride

supplements *only* for children age six months to 16 years living in non-fluoridated areas. The ADA acknowledges that children are exposed to additional ingested fluoride from other sources in everyday life—bottled water, fruits and vegetables, the water supply in places other than their home, beverages processed with fluoridated water and numerous other sources—but still recommends dosing these children with the preset "Fluoride Supplement Dosage Schedule-1994" as approved by themselves. The American Academy of Pediatrics and the American Academy of Pediatric Dentistry use dosage tables based upon the ADA recommendations; they do not do their own evaluation for dosage levels. This dosage is to be administered without even knowing whether a child might already be grossly overdosed with fluoride in the course of their everyday lives.

Yet even as early as 1994, members of the ADA were in disagreement about the use of dietary fluoride supplements. In an abstract given at the ADA Dietary Fluoride Supplement Conference that year, Dr. Brian Burt recommended discontinuance of these supplements because of the risk of overdosage and the studies showing no decay preventive action.

Prenatal Vitamins and Fluoride Effects

It was sometimes the practice to recommend to expectant mothers that they take daily doses of prenatal vitamins containing fluoride, presumably to prevent tooth decay in the unborn. The use of fluoride prenatal vitamins in a study by the Medical College of Georgia in Augusta, involved 1400 pregnant women in their first trimester of pregnancy. The study ended when the child reached the age of five. It was found that fluoride supplements had *no* beneficial effect on the tooth decay of the children evaluated at age three and five years.

Fluoride Toothpaste for General Use

As we've already seen, the ADA seal of approval is worth millions of dollars in sales to manufacturers of certain products. This has been especially true since the inception of toothpastes containing fluoride in the 1940s and 1950s. At that time there was considerable debate over allowing fluoride to be added to dentifrices for general public use. In the mid 1950s Colgate began producing a fluoride toothpaste. Its competitor Unilever introduced fluoridated Pepsodent and Procter & Gamble introduced Crest. Between 1954 and 1959 Procter & Gamble paid Indiana University enormous research dollars for studies to demonstrate the effectiveness of Crest with Fluoride in reducing cavities. After much lobbying, Crest toothpaste was given the American Dental Association's seal of approval in 1960 and its sales shot through the roof.

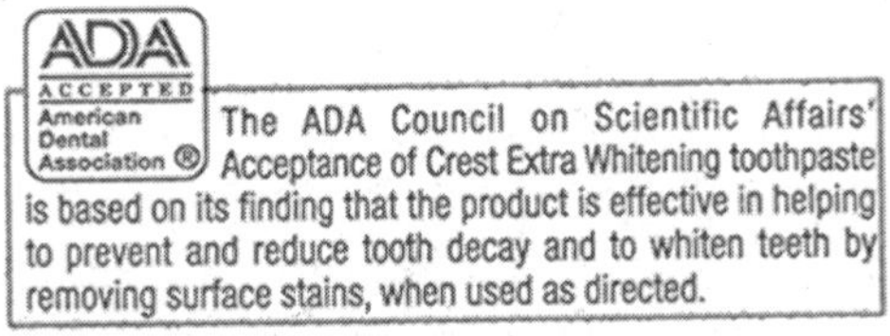

From the start, the ADA didn't give its seal of endorsement to fluoridated toothpaste and topical fluorides only for public health reasons—

The ADA Council on Scientific Affairs' Acceptance of Crest Extra Whitening toothpaste is based on its finding that the product is effective in helping to prevent and reduce tooth decay and to whiten teeth by removing surface stains, when used as directed.

Figure 3-7: The ADA seal of approval

and that isn't it's motive today either. The Association went as far as to recommend the use of a fluoride-containing toothpaste for everyone over the age of two years. Almost 50 years later, almost all toothpastes with fluoride carry the ADA seal.

The ADA contradicts itself, however, when it comes to exactly how much fluoride it recommends. By 1994 research showed environmental exposure to ingested fluoride by children was much higher than originally thought. Most children were being overexposed and overdosed with fluoride, some at toxic levels. The ADA backed down from its original position and revised its recommendations so no fluoride supplements should be used by children under six years of age. But if this trade association was concerned that as little as 0.25 mg of fluoride would harm these children, *why did it not reveal that brushing three times per day with a fluoride toothpaste allows ingestion of fluoride by the child of over 2 mg?* This approaches a severely toxic dose of fluoride for children.

Fluoride toothpaste should not be used. Period. But even when it is used, fluoride-containing toothpaste should never be used before a child is two years of age because of the very real danger of she or he swallowing the stuff. Statistics from the American Association of Poison Control Centers indicate how many poison control emergency calls are placed each year and for what drug or product.

Emergency calls to the American Association of Poison Control Center for ingestion of (swallowing) toothpaste containing fluoride:

♦ On average, over 22,000 calls are logged in each year.

♦ An average of 20,000 calls for emergencies to children under six years of age are reported each year.

♦ About 400 are treated in a health care facility.

♦ Only one death each year is recorded.

These statistics do *not* take into account the "non-calls," when children are sickened but the parent does not realize the danger and doesn't call for help. For ingestion of non-fluoride containing toothpaste, less than 1800 calls were made and 30 visits to health care facilities are noted.

Toothpaste containing fluoride is clearly a major source of fluoride overdose and toxicity. In 1994 the American Dental Association and American Academy of Pediatric Dentistry changed their recommendations to reflect this danger. A child under six years of age has difficulty with their swallowing reflex, and this is more pronounced under three years of age. And children are especially prone to swallow toothpaste if they like the flavor.

A child-sized toothbrush covered with a full strip of toothpaste holds approximately 0.75 to 1.0 gm of toothpaste, which at the over-the-counter toothpaste concentration of 1,500 ppm which comes out to approximately 1.0 mg of fluoride. A child under six years-of-age swallows about 0.3 gm of toothpaste each brushing, or can swallow as much as 0.8 mg of fluoride. *This could be as much as 2.4 mg fluoride per day, a fluoride overdose by any calculation!* (Using the chart on page 196, you can determine the amount of fluoride that is toxic according to the weight of the child.) The result has been that the CDC's recommendations were changed in 1991 to assure that children of less than two years of age used no fluoride toothpaste and those of less than six years used only a controlled amount of fluoride toothpaste. Their exact recommendation is to allow these two- to six-year-old children to use only a "pea size" amount of toothpaste on their brush. They are to be directed to spit out the paste and *not swallow any.* The FDA has also mandated the labeling requirements to reflect the danger of this toothpaste. So why, reader, do you constantly see advertisements for toothpaste in which the brush is depicted as *covered* with at least a one-inch length of paste? Are they trying to help our children or just sell as much toothpaste as possible? And where is the ADA *after* the famous Seal of Approval is given? Surely they insure that the manufacturers live up to the "standards" they themselves have set? They do not.

Yet it's also likely that most dentists conduct minimal discussions of these warnings and dangers with the parents of young children. And anyway, most dentists don't know how much toothpaste or gel or rinse is a probable lethal dose of fluoride for a child. Dental students are taught very little about the risks of fluoride ingestion. What actually *is* the "pea-size" amount of toothpaste mentioned by the ADA and the CDC to be used by children under six years of age? Is it not a highly subjective, visually-determined amount that could vary between any two parents? Peas vary dramatically in size, as you can see by visiting the frozen food section of any supermarket. What about the advice not to dispense "more than used for brushing"? How much is *that* amount and how does a parent know when "that amount" is reached? When the child gets sick or throws up? How harmless is a toothpaste if the FDA requires a poison control center be contacted if "too much" is ingested?

These pastes and rinses are *not* harmless. The ADA has done a disservice to the public by not disclosing the dangers. In fact, in 2006, they indirectly encouraged *overdoses* of fluoride by children. In their own publication, "ADA Statement Commemorating the 60th Anniversary of Community Water Fluoridation," they state, under Question 26, that a tube of toothpaste does not contain enough fluoride to seriously harm a child if ingested. *This is a blatant lie!*

The Food and Drug Administration *requires* a warning label on the fluoride toothpaste tube. (See Figure 3-9. page 217.) The public response by the ADA to regulations requiring a warning is that the ADA considers it too scary ("unnecessarily frightening") for people to know about possible fluoride poisoning. They contend that "the label overstates any demonstrated or potential danger posed by fluoride toothpastes." Apparently the FDA does not agree with them.

Just for the Kiddies

Well, the good folks who make toothpaste know they must be careful. That's why they produce special toothpastes for our children: those cute little squeeze bottles on

> Most toothpastes marketed for children contain the same concentration of fluoride as adult fluoride toothpastes.

the shelves in our supermarkets, the ones full of toothpaste in special kid's flavors like strawberry or bubble gum. Who wouldn't want to buy "Kids Colgate"? It's almost like candy, except it's "good" for our children. (Figure 3-10, p. 217)

Alas, the concentration of fluoride in this kid's toothpaste is about 1,100 parts per million, similar to that in a regular adult fluoride toothpaste. As far back as 1987, G.M. Whitford and many others established the Probable Toxic Dose (PTD) of fluoride to be 5 mg of fluoride per 1 kg of body weight. Above this level, a person could experience severe toxic consequences including emergency hospitalization, coma and death. Death is, in fact, likely at 15 milligrams per kilogram.

> If you still use fluoride toothpastes, keep them out of the reach
> of children and never allow children under eight to use them!

Look at the chart opposite, for which I'm grateful to www.fluoridealert.org. The 5.5-ounce size of the Colgate for Kids bottle contains 143 milligrams of fluoride. The chart, based on the average weight of children at various ages, shows what percentage of the bottle, if swallowed, is required to kill your child.

Minimum Lethal Dose of Fluoride Contained in One Tube of "Colgate for Kids" Toothpaste			
Age of Child	Average Weight*	Dose of fluoride which could kill child	Percent of "Colgate for Kids" toothpaste which. if swallowed. could kill child**
2 years	~12 kg	60 mg	42% of tube
3 years	~15 kg	75 mg	53%, of tube
4 years	~16 kg	80 mg¹	56% of tube
5 years	~18 kg	90 mg	63% of tube
6 years	~20 kg	100 mg	70% of tube
7 years	~22 kg	110 mg	77% of tube
8 years	~25 kg	125 mg	87% of tube
9 years	~28 kg	140 mg	98% of tube
*Average weight data obtained here			
** The fluoride concentration in Colgate for Kids toothpaste is 1,100 ppm. At 130 gm of paste in the average tube, this equals 143 mg of fluoride.			

Table 3-3: Lethal dose of toothpaste per age and weight of child (courtesy Fluoride Action Network)

As you can see, if your average 3-year-old weighing 15 kg or 33 lb swallows ½ of this bottle, he or she will ingest 72 mg of fluoride and almost certainly fall deathly sick, probably fall into a coma, and possibly die. There is no antidote after the fluoride is ingested and absorbed in the stomach. Dialysis might be tried as a last resort.

Many parents have child-proofed their homes. They put plastic blanks in the electric outlets, put dangerous chemical cleaners and solvents high above a child's reach, place child locks on

> Most toothpastes marketed for children contain the same concentration of fluoride as adult fluoride toothpastes.

kitchen and bathroom cabinets. Then they leave the tube of fluoride toothpaste sitting on the bathroom counter, with a flavor designed to entice small children.

Fluoride in Toothpastes: Actual Numbers

So here is the information you must know, presented as simply as I can.

♦ One part per million of fluoride in your drinking water is equal to 1 mg of fluoride in 1 quart of water.

♦ One tube of average adult fluoride toothpaste contains about 1,100 ppm of fluoride, with toothpastes ranging from 500 to 1,500 ppm.

♦ An average large tube contains 7.8 oz (221 grams) of toothpaste or a total of 243 mg of fluoride. An average 3-year-old weighing 15 kg/33 lb would only need to swallow or eat 30% of the toothpaste in this tube to have a life-threatening reaction.

♦ Sodium fluoride (NaF) is often used in dental products. One milligram of NaF is equal to 0.45 milligrams of fluoride.

♦ The active ingredient in most fluoride toothpastes, NaF, is present in the same concentration whether for child or adult consumption. Don't be fooled by the size of the tube, bottle or box. If it looks

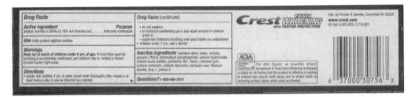

Figure 3-11: Adult-size tube of fluoride toothpaste

about the same size when put on a toothbrush, it has the same amount of fluoride in it.

AGAIN:

Drinking Water: 1 ppm F = 1 mg fluoride per 1 quart water
Toothpaste: one large tube = 1,100 ppm F = 243 mg fluoride (listed on box as 0.243% sodium fluoride)
Most toothpastes marketed for children contain the same concentration of fluoride as adult fluoride toothpastes.

Washout: Fluoride Rinses for Caries-Prone Patients

Fluoride rinses have been rec-ommended by the ADA for dental patients with unique dental care needs. Most den-tists believe what they were told in dental school: If a little fluoride can prevent tooth decay, high doses of fluoride will stop decay and tooth sen-sitivity even more effectively. Patients who demonstrate ex-cessive tooth decay, even

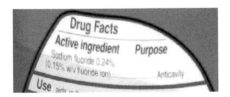

Figure 3-12: The concentration of fluoride listed on the bottle label of this well-known fluoride toothpaste for children is the same as the adult concentration.

with full dental prophylactic measures taken by the dental team, are subject to recommendations of ancillary fluoride use through home-use rinses or gels.

The concentration of fluoride in these home products is very high. Whereas normal fluoride toothpaste has fluoride concentrations of 1,000 to 1500 ppm, fluoride rinses and gels can have 5,000 ppm or more. The FDA allows them to be recommended only on the prescription by a licensed doctor. But if fluoride is so harmless, why is it by prescription only? *Because improper or excessive use of the gel or rinse exposes the person to toxic levels of fluoride and potential health risks.*

The rationale for home-use fluoride rinses and gels is the same as for topical fluoride treatments in the dental office. Dentists believe fluoride will exert its anti-cavity and anti-tooth-sensitivity actions immediately and then with residual effects over time—hours or days with regular and continuous use. Yet carefully conducted studies have demonstrated over and over that fluoride is effective *only* while it is present on the surface of the tooth. It is the actual *presence* of fluoride in the mouth and saliva that inhibits the protein metabolism of the bacteria that produce the acids that cause tooth decay. In the mouth, if fluoride is present at all, it is soon washed away with normal saliva flow and certainly if the person drinks or eats anything. Since it is present only very superficially in tooth structure, there is no residual fluoride remaining to protect anything.

Fluoride for Sensitive Teeth: the Hype

Patients with generalized tooth sensitivity are also placed on home fluoride use. Generalized tooth sensitivity usually means sensitivity causing mild to severe pain triggered by:

♦ Consuming cold or hot liquids or foods
♦ Cold air breathed in through the mouth
♦ Brushing teeth, mostly at the gum line
♦ Eating certain foods like sweets or acidic foods
♦ Chewing on or grinding the teeth together
♦ Touching the tooth where it meets the gum line.

Most tooth sensitivity is caused by recession of the gingiva (attached gum) away from the neck of the tooth. This recession uncovers tooth root surface that was previously covered and protected. Most people think of a tooth as solid and without nerves except for the main nerve canal in the middle. Actually, although the enamel that covers the exposed part of the tooth is solid and with no surface innervation,

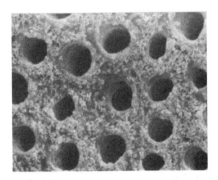

Figure 3-13: Nerve tubules opening onto the root surface (organic tissue removed)

the root structure below the healthy gingival level has millions of microscopic canals or channels called dentinal tubules. These tubules hold extensions of the central nerve from the core through the root structure and out onto the surface of the root within the bony tooth socket itself. These nerve extensions are exposed to the air when the gums recede, and so cause the pain when stimulated.

Ever since the ADA gave their "seal of approval" to manufacturers for fluoridated toothpastes and topical fluoride office treatments, manufacturers have tried to promote fluoride as a desensitizing medication for these patients. It's not entirely clear why the fluoride presence on the surface of the exposed root decreases tooth sensitivity in some patients. Most theories suggest the fluoride somehow blocks the openings of the dentinal tubules so the nerves coming onto the root surface are

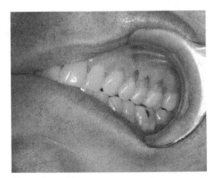

Figure 3-14: Abfractions causing gum recession

inaccessible. Since fluoride has been shown to only be effective while in the saliva and mouth, it is reasonable to suspect that fluoride blocking these tubules is eventually washed away. This would explain why patients' sensitivity returns within so short a time after treatment and why the effectiveness of blocking the tubules may not work at all with some patients, who get no relief from their tooth sensitivity through use of additional fluoride rinses and gels.

When people use these prescribed high-concentration fluoride gels and rinses, they're exposed to levels of fluoride five times or more higher than those received through use of routine fluoride toothpastes. The instructions given for use of these products vary from manufacturer to manufacturer and from dentist to dentist. Generally patients are told to floss and brush their teeth as usual, then apply the gel to the roots of the sensitive teeth or, if it comes as a rinse, to just swish a certain amount around in their mouth for a period of time, usually a couple of minutes. Then they must spit it out and try not to swallow any. They must not eat or drink anything for at least 30 minutes. Of course: *fluoride only works topically against both tooth decay and sensitive roots.* It is soon washed away from the teeth and mouth with normal swallowing of saliva and any foods or beverages. And as we're about to see, swallowing the high concentrations of fluoride in the solutions can be hazardous to your health.

Many home or over-the-counter products claim to reduce tooth sensitivity, some combined with fluoride in the product and some without fluoride. Some are effective and some not. Some may contain toxic components that are potentially dangerous, especially to children. Others do not. Be careful to examine the labels. Fluoride may not be the only ingredient to cause health concerns. Beside fluoride, artificial sweeteners like saccharin (metabolism disturbances) or sorbitol (laxative effects in some adults and children) or sodium bicarbonate (salts are contraindicated for high blood pressure or heart problems) are undesirable.

Tooth sensitivity may be caused by factors other than root exposure. Patients with a recent dental filling that was not completely adjusted for their bite (occlusion) may find that the tooth hits the opposite tooth when they bite before their other teeth make contact. This premature contact every time the patient closes or bites his or her teeth together causes inflammation around the tooth socket, which in turn causes sensitivity. This type of sensitivity is not helped by procedures to seal the root surface, but can only be rectified by adjusting the bite on the offending tooth so it and the other teeth make simultaneous contact with their opposing teeth. Relief of the excessive pressure usually reduces or eliminates any sensitivity.

The Poison Apples

Snow White almost died because the apple looked so good. Many things in our modern world masquerade as good for us when in reality they're dangerous. Some—the big, fat cheeseburger, for example—are minor dangers. Others—thalidomide, for example, a supposedly safe drug taken during pregnancy to help the mother sleep better, turned out to have incredibly sinister effects: hundreds of catastrophic birth defects.

That's why I keep urging you to look closely at things recommended to you—especially dental and medical prescriptions and products such as high-level fluorides for tooth sensitivity. Do your own research. If you have children, you must look out for them too.

The consensus among those researchers and clinicians who see cases of fluoride overdoses in children, is that today's child is already exposed to vast amounts of fluoride in their foods and beverages. It wasn't so 40 years ago and these researchers believe that prescribing additional dietary fluoride supplements is not warranted. They advise that clinicians and dentists exercise caution in prescribing fluoride and to do so only in extreme cases of rampant uncontrolled decay. Excess fluoride, as we're beginning to see, can have severe dental and health consequences.

As packaged, many dental products have quantities of fluoride that can exceed the probable toxic dose (PTD) of 5 mg per kg of body weight of your child. *One scary study by Levy in the 1994 Community Dentistry and Oral Epidemiology journal, demonstrated that 85% of both pediatric and general dentists did not know the correct age to begin and end fluoride supplements. Only 6% of those dentists who responded to the survey routinely tested the fluoride level in the drinking water of the patient before prescribing supplements.* This essential and thorough testing is even recommended by the ADA and the American Academy of Pediatrics.

The amount of fluoride in dental products used at home is actually increasing. This has an impact on children and small adults who unknowingly ingest certainly lethal doses of fluoride. Amounts as low as 5 gm of sodium fluoride can cause death in a 70 kg (154 lb) person. Only 1 to 1.25 gm may be ingested maximally as a safely tolerated dose. Even greater caution must be taken in light of the excessive amounts of fluoride already in the child's diet and toothpaste.

Fluoridation of the Water Supply

Early on in this chapter, I recounted the story of fluoride's introduction into our water supply, a process in which the dentistry profession has played a significant role. Today, the United States is one of only a few countries worldwide to add fluoride to its drinking water.

In recent news, the ADA and the public health services have tried to fluoridate the public water supply in a number of communities, including Yardley, York and Shaler in Pennsylvania, Juneau in Alaska, and Quebec City in Canada. They have been voted down in public referendums over the last few years. When presented with the overwhelming evidence of the toxic effects of fluoride, these communities understood the dangers and refused the mandatory fluoridation. Since 1990 over 150 communities have voted down community fluoridation.

On August 9, 2007, the US Centers for Disease Control received a formal complaint for ethics violations in connection with information not released on fluoride cautions. The CDC did not release the findings by the US National Research Council that kidney patients, diabetics, infants and seniors are especially susceptible to harm from fluoride.

Other Sources of Fluoride

Aside from dental- and oral-care products and the fluoridated water supply—all of which have received general support from the dental profession—there are many other sources of fluoride exposure.

♦ Foods and beverages manufactured or bottled in cities with fluoridated water. (See section on fluoride in drinking water, page 203.) The FDA published data showing fluoride concentration in bottled water can range from 1.4 to 2.4 ppm depending on the outside air temperatures where the water was bottled.

♦ Fluoride–containing pesticide residues in food. The US EPA is considering letting the DOW Chemical Company use Vikane™ gas (sulfuryl fluoride), a 1950s structural fumigant used to kill insects and pests, to fumigate *food processing plants and warehouses.* If allowed this will leave a fluoride residue on our food supply as the levels permitted would be huge: 900 ppm in powdered eggs and 130 ppm in wheat flour.

♦ Other medical products and medicines that contain fluoride and fluoride compounds.

♦ Ocean air and fish can contain 1.4 ppm fluoride.

♦ Shower steam and humidifiers using fluoridated water.

♦ Fluoride in foods (e.g., tea, vegetables grown in fluoridated communities).

A Safe Level of Fluoride

It's important to realize that these alarming views on the poisonous potential of fluoride compounds are not those held by some militant fringe of toxin zealots, as the media once loved to paint it. The zealotry, if anywhere, has been on the other side. The mass of scientific consensus has moved steadily against what many still complacently regard as good public health policy.

The natural, healthy human body contains only a trace amount of fluoride. Breast milk contains 0.024–0.172 mg/L. More than that must be considered excessive. Though many doctors still prescribe dietary fluoride supplements that are from 0.25 mg for an 18-month to three-year-old up to 1 mg for six- to 12-year-olds, established medical researchers and scientific investigators have now reached a consensus: everyday exposure to fluoride in the average child's environment and diet *exceeds all recommended daily allowances* for maximum fluoride exposures. This overexposure can be dangerously close to the levels causing serious health consequences due to excessive fluoride.

In 1997 the National Academy of Science (NAS) published a dietary reference book for fluoride. The data they released claimed the following levels of total ingested fluoride that would not cause dental fluorosis, dental fluorosis being their indicator for the earliest sign of excess fluoride exposure.

♦ *Infants (under six months)* should get no more than *0.01 mg per day*. This is hard to achieve because most foods contain more than that amount. Fluoride concentrations were measured when infant formula powder was mixed with three types of water. Readings were 0.01–0.75 mg/L with distilled water, 0.02–1.37 mg/L with bottled water, and 0.91–1.55 mg/L with fluoridated tap water. As you can see from these levels, only those formulas mixed with pure distilled water could possibly stay below the limit of fluoride exposure.

> If you reconstitute infant powdered formula with water for an infant less than six months old, use only distilled water.

♦ *Babies (six–12 months)* should get under *0.5 mg daily*. Again this is difficult to stay below because most foods will supply more than that level of fluoride. For example, a single serving of mechanically separated and pureed chicken baby food (a 2.5 oz serving) may by itself contain 0.6 mg of fluoride. Infant foods had the highest fluoride content, followed by chicken sticks, luncheon meats and canned meats. Foods made with turkey were not a significant source of fluoride.

♦ *Toddlers (one–three years)* must stay below *0.7 mg daily*. Yet some milk varieties alone have 0.72 mg/L of fluoride.

♦ *Young Children (four–eight years)* may not exceed *1 mg per day*. Fruit Loops™ have measured 2.1 mg/L of fluoride.

The American Dental Association has now reduced its recommended levels of fluoride and even agreed that practitioners should review a patient's fluoride levels from all sources before adding further to that patient's fluoride burden. But truly well informed dentists will examine *all* the evidence and know that fluoride should never be prescribed in the first place.

The American Academy of Pediatrics published an article as early as 1998 revealing that even pediatricians teaching in medical center facilities did not follow treatment recommendations for prescribing oral fluoride supplements. Only 70% of these doctors determined the fluoride content of the child's drinking water before prescribing supplements. Less than 87% knew the correct dosage for children of various ages. Only 58% referred their patients for routine dental examination and care before they were three years of age. This is all contrary to recommendations by the American Academy of Pediatrics. These doctors are supposed to represent the most knowledgeable of medical personnel prescribing fluoride supplementation, yet *many were ignorant of the protocols intended to avoid serious health consequences.*

In a 1987 edition of the *Journal of Dental Research*, G.M. Whitford advanced the concept of a "certain lethal dose" (CLD) as compared to a "probable toxic dose" (PTD). The certain lethal dose range for a 70 kg (154 lb) adult is from 5 to 10 grams of sodium fluoride, equal to 2.25 to 4.54 grams of actual fluoride. If this adult ingests 2.5 grams (2500 mg) of actual fluoride, in any form, he or she will probably die. Whitford defined the probable toxic dose as the dose of "ingested fluoride that should trigger immediate therapeutic intervention and hospitalization because of...serious toxic consequences." This PTD, or, in effect, the minimum lethal dose, is listed as 5.0 mg of fluoride per kg of body weight. A 70-kg man who ingests 350 mg of fluoride, will be going to the hospital. These levels of toxic fluoride are fairly high and an adult is unlikely to reach them by accident. Whitford, however, evaluated dental products and their levels of contained fluoride and concludes that "most of them exceed the PTD [of fluoride] for young children." He recommended reduction in the use of products that may exceed toxic levels if taken in combinations or excess. The Canadian Dental Association, in 2000, advised against fluoride supplementation before the age of six or seven, when the permanent teeth start to erupt. Many countries have banned the use of products containing fluoride altogether. In 2002, Belgium banned the use of tablets and chewing gum that contain fluoride in response to fears that these products increase the risk of brittle bone disease. Under the Code of Federal Regulations of the US Food and Drug Administration (FDA), a warning must be put on the label of all fluoridated products:

> I. (1) *For all fluoride dentifrice (gel, paste, and powder) products.*
> "Keep out of reach of children under six years of age. [highlighted in bold type] If more than used for brushing is accidentally swallowed, get medical help or contact a Poison Control Center right away." These warnings shall be used in place of the general warning statements required by 330.1 (g) of this chapter.

> II. (2) *For all fluoride rinse and preventive treatment gel products.*
> "Keep out of reach of children. [highlighted in bold type] If

more than used for" (select appropriate word: "brushing" or "rinsing") "is accidentally swallowed, get medical help or contact a Poison Control Center right away." These warnings shall be used in place of the general warning statements required by 330.1(g) of this chapter.

—FDA required warning on fluoride product

The Shell Game

"C'mon! How long has fluoride been around? So how come we haven't heard anything about how dangerous it is?"

Man, I wish I had a dollar for every time I've heard that one, from dentists and laypersons alike. I understand how difficult it is to accept as untrue a story you've been told for years and accepted as true. I myself felt just like that about Santa Clause and the Easter Bunny. And cigarettes. How long did we hear and believe that cigarette smoking was harmless to our health? How many painters scoffed at the claims that lead in paint damaged mental functioning?

The shell game was for centuries a perennial favorite among street flimflam men. As passers-by looked on, the fellow would set up three half walnut shells on a flat surface, usually something like a wooden milk crate. He'd take a pea and place it under one of the shells, shuffle the shells back and forth and around the table, sliding them to and fro with both hands for several seconds as the onlookers tried to follow the one hiding the pea. He would then ask the onlookers to wager a bet. "Which shell is the pea under?" If the bettor guessed correctly, the shuffler would pay the bet even money. If the shuffler was honest, he had a two-to-one chance of winning. If he was a skilled shuffler, his odds were hugely increased. But if the shuffler was dishonest, he could use slight-of-hand to remove the pea from play while sliding the shells. The bettor would have no chance whatsoever. The crooked shuffler relied upon the bettors not knowing what was really going on. He controlled the game and the outcome.

When I learned about fluoride concentrations in dental school, even I could not explain or easily calculate the exact relationship between the amounts of fluoride in foods, water, dietary tablets, toothpastes and fluoride gels. The units of measure were elusively incompatible. How did parts per million relate to grams of fluoride in a topical gel? How did 1 mg of oral fluoride supplement relate to swallowing too much toothpaste? By not giving the public the whole story, fluoride suppliers, manufacturers of dental products containing fluoride, and the American Dental Association could trick the public into accepting their "expert conclusions." The pea—the recognition that for decades children were getting too much fluoride and that adults didn't need it added to their water—was kept out of the game.

FLUORIDE: THE ALTERNATIVES

Whenever I speak to a group about the hazards of fluoride, I'm met with skeptical and disbelieving eyes. We've been told for over 50 years about the supposed benefits of fluoride and, as we've seen over and over, change is hard. Doctors don't like to change beliefs and procedures they're comfortable with, and neither does the general public. It's comforting to believe there's a substance out there, a magic

> There are now alternatives to fluoride's mythical qualities that it is truly safe, effective and healthy...products that actually provide more protection for children and adults than fluoride was supposed to do.

bullet, that can stop tooth decay and tooth sensitivity and all we have to do is *use it*. But the troubling truth is that we must look at everything we put into our bodies with both eyes open. We must question not only the benefits but the unfortunate downsides as well. We must conduct a constant balancing act to weigh the pros

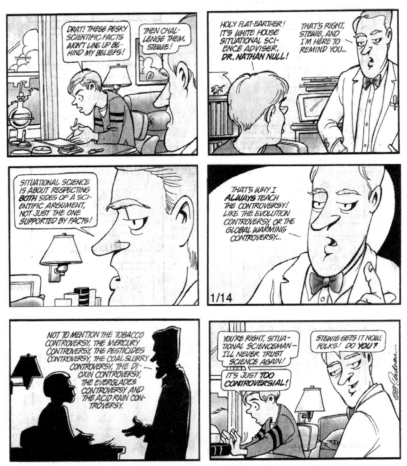

Figure 3-15: DOONESBURY © 2006 G. B. Trudeau. Reprinted with permission of UNIVERSAL PRESS SYNDICATE. All rights reserved

against the cons and decide if the perceived benefit is worth a health risk.

What do we do when the negatives are not revealed? Through no fault of our own, the negatives about fluoride have been covered up since fluoride was first introduced as a decay-preventive supplement. I assure you I cannot help but feel paranoid when I preach the hazards of fluoride poisoning to a people who have never been exposed to the research.

I will tell them the same thing I tell my patients: don't believe me. Believe your own inquiry. The Internet is a fantastic equalizer. Yes, there are plenty of whacko websites out there, but you'll soon learn to identify authoritative sources and respected institutions' sites. Governments can tell lie after lie about their actions and corporations can tell lie after lie about their products, but these days, the truth sooner or later appears on the Internet! Please confirm what you have been reading here with documents readily available on the web. At first, you'll probably become angry that one of the biggest hoaxes in the history of medicine and dentistry was pulled on the North American public. Next, you'll feel outrage that the health of the public—ordinary people such as you and your children—was put in jeopardy. And then—as I hope—you'll be motivated to do something about this attack. We must all become politically active to *get fluoride out of our lives.*

I'm certainly *not* asking you to abandon your efforts to prevent tooth decay or gum disease. Given what we now know about the ineffectiveness of fluoride as an anti-caries agent, you may well be concerned about how to prevent tooth decay and periodontal disease. When I first realized the dangers of using any fluoride-containing product and eliminated all these from my practice, I was faced with a quandary. This was many years ago and the only alternatives to fluoride toothpastes were simple dentifrices—cleaning agents such as peppermint oil and baking soda. These products did a good job of cleaning the surfaces of the teeth off, but people were used to having a toothpaste that fought decay. I too viewed these simple dentifrices as a step back in dental history. But I preached what I knew to be true: good oral hygiene and home care, and a reasonable diet, wins out against decay.

Thank God for independent dental research! There are now alternatives to fluoride's mythical qualities that are truly safe, effective and healthy. Some of these products actually provide more protection for children and adults than fluoride was supposed to do. They can restore damaged teeth surfaces, fight tooth decay and reduce and eliminate tooth or root sensitivity. And your young child can swallow the contents of a tube and not be deathly sick. All you need do is investigate and choose the alternative that works for you.

Fighting Tooth Decay and Sensitive Teeth

There are several alternative active ingredients and some of these are incorporated into certain toothpastes and rinses. The current dental hygiene emphasis is on *remineralization of the tooth surface*. Tooth decay and open exposure of the microscopic dentinal tubules in the root surfaces are the targets for these products. Three of the compounds use a form of calcium phosphate and the fourth uses a combination of an amino acid and calcium. They are:

♦ Arginine bicarbonate/calcium carbonate
♦ Amorphous calcium phosphate
♦ Calcium peroxide/carbamide peroxide/activators
♦ Calcium/phosphorus/silica/sodium particles.

I'm going to describe four products. The list is, by the very nature of research and development, incomplete as new products are constantly emerging. You *must* know the active ingredients you are looking for and read the labels of all home products you buy.

1. Arginine Bicarbonate/Calcium Carbonate (CaviStat®)

Marketed as Denclude™ and Proclude® by Ortek Therapeutics, Inc. (now owned by the Colgate-Palmolive Company).

This combination of compounds work individually and together. Arginine is an amino acid normally found in the human body. When applied to the teeth, plaque bacteria that produce decay-forming acids break down the arginine bicarbonate into alkaline (base pH) products. These alkaline products neutralize the acids to prevent decalcification of the tooth surface and stop the subsequent tooth decay. The calcium carbonate counters any dissolution of the tooth surface and helps remineralize (recalcify) the tooth.

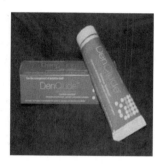

Figure 3-16: Denclude toothpaste

Ortek Therapeutics has researched and verified this action over a 2-year study of 11- to 12-year-olds, and published the results in the *Journal of Clinical Dentistry*.

Both products (Denclude™ and Proclude®) have been the subject of verified research that shows up to a 90% reduction in tooth sensitivity for up to 28 days with Proclude® and a 60% reduction for Denclude™. Their proprietary ingredients are marketed under the name *SensiStat*™.

The Denclude™ toothpaste is safe to use for all ages. Under FDA regulations, it is available only on the order of a dentist. The Proclude® prophylaxis paste is used by dentists and hygienists during routine dental office polishings.

Neither contains fluoride. However when I spoke to their research scientists, they told me they had to add a small amount of saccharin to improve the taste. In my opinion, of all the synthetic sugar substitutes, none of which I personally use, a small amount of saccharin in the toothpaste is the least likely to be harmful.

2. Amorphous Calcium Phosphate (ACP)

Marketed as Arm & Hammer Enamel Care® Toothpaste

This is a 2-phase delivery system. The toothpaste tube has two compartments which mix their contents as the paste is expressed onto the toothbrush. One has the calcium and the other the phosphate. The mixing together activates the components to form active

ACP. The ACP dissolves in the saliva and the calcium released re-mineralizes the tooth surface.

The only scientific study supporting claims for this product is that for the fluoride in the mix. The claim is for reduced dental decay.

This combination has great potential but cannot be recommended at this time because *it contains fluoride.*

3. Casein Phosphopeptide and Amorphous Calcium Phosphate (CPP-ACP)

Marketed as Recaldent™ in Trident White® Sugarless Gum (Cadbury Adams USA) and in Prospec™ MI paste (GC America, Inc).

Casein phosphopeptide (CPP) is a protein found in milk. The gum consists of a coating of CPP over the ACP.

The anticariogenic potential of CPP-ACP has been attributed to the ability of the CPP to localize amorphous calcium phosphate at the tooth surface, that is, help the complex stick to the tooth surface. The acid produced by the plaque bacteria releases the ACP, which adheres to and is absorbed into the tooth surface. This helps to maintain a state of supersaturation with respect to the tooth mineral and thus remineral-izes the tooth surface.

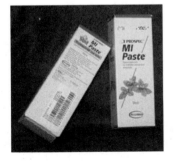

Bonlac Foods Ltd, the company producing Recalcant, claims it also re-duces tooth sensitivity.

There is evidence the molecule may wash away quickly from the tooth sur-face before it is absorbed. This would lead to recurrent sensitivity sooner

Figure 3-17: MI Paste toothpaste

than desired. One study showed Recalcant does not block the den-tinal tubules as well and for as long as the modified bioglass material such as NovaMin®. These products contain no fluoride.

4. Calcium/Phosphorus/Silica/Sodium Particle

Marketed as NovaMin®, as Oravive Tooth Revitalizing Paste (Oravive), Soothe Rx® (Omni Pharmaceuticals/3M) and as Butler NuCare™ Tooth Root Conditioner (Sunstar Butler).

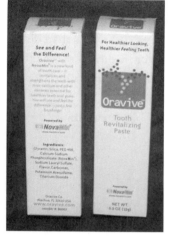

The four elements—calcium, phosphorus, silica and sodium—occur naturally in the body. When the NovaMin® particles contact saliva or water, they release the sodium, phosphorus and calcium ions that are then available for remineralization of the tooth surface. The claimed benefit of this product is the direct formation into the tooth of hydroxyapatite

Figure 3-18: Oravive Revitalizing Paste (contains NovaMin®)

(HAP), the form of mineral calcium that comprises tooth enamel structure. The other calcium phosphate products must first form a middle step, amorphous calcium phosphate, before being available to the tooth surface.

Research study has shown the mineral ions are available to the tooth structure up to two weeks after release.

NovaMin® has anti-microbial properties and can kill almost 100% of oral pathogens associated with periodontal disease and decay (caries). The company claims the Oravive® or SoothRx® toothpaste reduces gingivitis up to 58% used twice each day for six weeks.

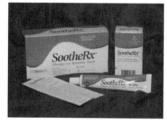

This product is approved by the FDA for treatment of tooth sensitivity

Figure 3-19; SootheRx® for sensitive teeth (contains NovaMin®)

and has great potential. It is extremely effective for this purpose and has a wealth of studies that all validate its performance. However in my opinion most of the research has gone into diminishing tooth sensitivity rather than developing anti-decay properties. NovaMin® *has* been shown to be effective in its antibacterial action.

It contains no fluoride.

A Last Hurrah

If you're feeling a little punch drunk from a stream of bad news, take heart. We'll look at just one more problem area—one that few people, even dentists, would suspect. And then we will give you help to find a dental practice that can truly make a difference in your overall health.

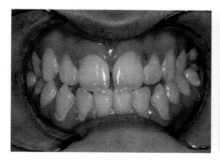
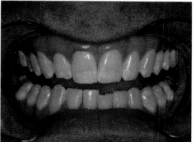

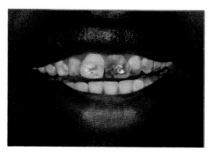

Figure 3-3: Dental fluorosis
from mild to extreme

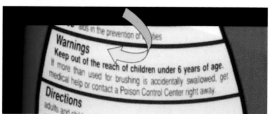

Figure 3-9: FDA warning about fluoride use
on every product containing fluoride

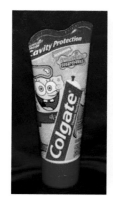
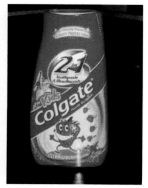

Figure 3-10: Colgate Toothpaste for Kids

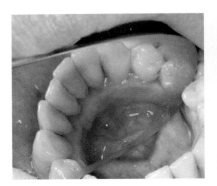

Figure 4-1: Calculus (tartar) inside lower front teeth can develop in a few months even if the patient is trying to brush properly. It takes time to remove these hard deposits.

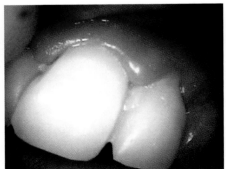

Figure 4-5: Full crowns on three teeth left no room for the gum tissue or floss. Acute ulcerating gingivitis resulted. Crowns had to be removed and remade. Permanent gum loss resulted.

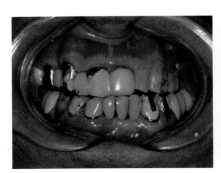

Figure 4-7: Over many years, gradual wear of old crowns is to be expected.

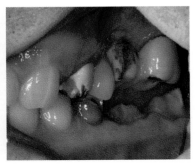

Figure 4-9: Porcelain too thin with poor bite causing porcelain to break away from underlying metal

4
TAKING CONTROL

**"I called my dentist back and he said he couldn't help
me."**

~ Tina Chen

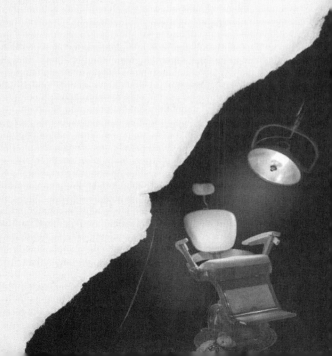

EXPECTATIONS, THEN AND NOW

The pace of our lives was slower 40 or 50 years ago, with less overall stress and time management. We were less distracted by recreational, business and entertainment preoccupations. There was no such thing as taking a laptop computer home and working all evening. People lived in the same neighborhoods all their lives and raised children who grew up and lived there too. They prepared meals in their own homes and ate out rarely. Their grocery stores were there, their doctors and dentists were there, their churches and temples were there. The streets were shady and lined with grass and trees. The traffic was sparse. Evenings were the long relaxing hours before bedtime.

At the same time, many people were health conscious in those days. You had to be alert to changes in your health because you could easily die from what are now treatable ailments. I myself was one of those children who missed school many times each year due to colds, flus and elevated temperatures of unknown origin. Dr. Wishnofsky was often called to our house. Dr. Wishnofsky was a sober and straightforward man of 52. He had a deep voice, a dedicated and authoritative manner and a genuine love of medicine. Whatever he said was accepted by us as absolute fact, as though conveyed directly from God through the medium of Dr. Wishnofsky's unprepossessing person. We believed that if we failed to follow his directions, the result might well be worsening health or death. We generally respected all our physicians as caregivers and healers, honest persons whose only concern was our health and well-being.

Ironically, even as late as the 1950s, there were real limitations on what a physician could offer. People died from medical conditions that are easily treated today. Only a generation earlier, influenza had killed tens of thousands of people each year. Polio was an ever-present threat. Simple colds were not simple. There were no vaccines or zeolite fourth generation of antibiotics. Hospital care could not improve the patient's condition unless surgery was needed, so most people were treated at home.

I'd see the dentist twice each year as a young child, as did the rest of my family. Our local dentist, Dr. Miller, had his office over a candy store, a location of outstanding convenience. The entrance was at street level. There was no elevator, just a narrow stairway ending in a frosted glass door plainly lettered in black, *Dr. David Miller, Dentist.* When you entered, you walked immediately into his waiting room. No matter what time of day, there were always people waiting to see Dr. Miller ahead of you. They were standing or seated, and were usually reading magazines, some so old that the pages were a mass of wrinkled sheets. No music played. There was no air conditioning in hot weather. There were no set appointments, so people just kept track of who was ahead of them when they walked in. The treatment room itself was behind another door of frosted glass with one of those glass doorknobs. You couldn't see through it but you could hear through it. We children awaited our turns with our parent as we listened to the whirrings and clickings, the moans and groans coming from the other side.

Finally—sometimes you waited an hour and a half—you went in. There was only one treatment room. It had a dental chair, equipment and enameled cabinets in black and white. Dr. Miller was a pleasant, unthreatening man who wore a white coat, a pair of black slacks and a perpetual smile. He was always chewing gum. Sugarless gum hadn't been invented yet. The room had an old x-ray unit in the corner behind the dental chair and a little closet off to the side in which he developed the x-rays. There was no assistant, hygienist or secretary. Dr. Miller performed all the procedures himself, including collecting his fee. It seemed like a simple profession.

When Dr. Miller took an x-ray, he'd hold it with his own fingers in my mouth and press the exposure button. The health risks of radiation were not widely recognized and doctors and dentists were often directly exposed to radiation. Then again, people didn't live quite as long as they do today, so maybe it didn't matter.

Dr. Miller drilled decay out of teeth without the bother of anesthesia. Hence the cries and moans. If the pain was too severe or the decay too deep, he'd extract the tooth. Only for that procedure would he inject the patient with anesthetic. To fill the tooth he used mercury amalgam. He'd mix a measured amount of liquid mercury from a glass bottle, with a dental alloy (a metal powder of silver, and copper or tin or zinc) in a ceramic mortar with a pestle. He inhaled the mercury vapor without reservation and so unwittingly exposed himself to severe toxicity. After he'd ground the mercury and alloy together, he'd dump the mercury-soaked filling material into his bare palm and roll it there with his bare fingers to complete the mixing. But the amalgam mix had to be as free as possible of liquid elemental mercury, so he'd put it on a small piece of cheesecloth and squeeze out the excess mercury between his fingers while his skin absorbed it freely. Only then did he pick up an instrument to start pushing the amalgam into the drilled tooth. Dr. Miller never saw any need for gloves. Even when immersed in blood during an extraction or handling the mercury, he never wore gloves. We have no mortality statistics for dentists in those days.

It's easy, with the advantage of hindsight, to smile at Dr. Miller's rough and ready approach to our safety—and his own. We naturally patronize the cozy memory of men like this, memories sometimes suffused with nostalgia. That's why it comes almost as a shock to realize that, in some important respects, we received better health care then than now.

How can I say that? Dr. Miller and Dr. Wishnofsky, as different as they were, had something fundamental in common. They were both caring, dedicated doctors who tried to do everything they could to help their patients. Neither one discussed with the patient the professional fees for their services *before* they were performed; their fees were assumed to be—known to be—reasonable. And in those days, there was no insurance coverage to discuss. Their motives for practicing were altruistic and noble in a strange way. If the patient didn't have the money to pay them for the services they performed, the patient would "owe" it to them. Trust was important on both sides of the doctor–patient relationship. Both our doctors were happy to make a comfortable living doing the job they loved.

Most doctors 50 years ago gave their patients the best information medical and dental science could provide. Yes, there were fewer diagnostic tools and tests available. There were fewer alternative treatments and almost no objective-outcomes research to recommend those alternatives. The number of drugs on the market at that time was nothing compared to the quantity available now. The big pharmaceutical companies hadn't begun their campaigns to convince doctors to treat patients with their company's products.

That was then. Unlike the practices of Drs. Miller and Wishnofsky, dental and medical practices today are *businesses*. They used to be *professions* but with the arrival of insurance companies and government regulations to manipulate the medical systems for their own purposes and profit, the true, caring doctors have a hard time swimming against the current to practice the way they would like—in the best interests of their patients.

"Sounds tough," you might say. "What's it got to do with *my* care?"

To start with, it has to do with how well you're treated in modern dental and medical offices. I spend a major portion of my time in administrative duties to run my practice. I'm lucky if I have enough time to treat patients. Unlike the doctors of yesteryear, I have a high monthly office expense and several employees that need to be paid. My bottom line at the end of the month is of as much concern to me as helping patients. If I don't make money, I won't be around to treat patients. If I don't make money, I can't keep up with improvements in my field. If I don't make money, I can't buy new equipment to perform procedures more safely and effectively. Who wants a doctor with old, worn furniture in the waiting room? Who wants a doctor who employs old, worn treatments and equipment? And by the way, who will put money away for my retirement if not me?

The average number of patients seen by a US physician is 12 per hour.
How can you, the patient, get a thorough evaluation and treatment
in a five-minute appointment? Yet if a physician is getting only a
tenth of his fee from a medical HMO, how can he spend more time
with a patient? In the US, many people simply don't know that
most doctors must write off the balance of their fees after the small
payment from the insurance company. They never see the rest.

A further factor in less than optimal care is, alas, professional arro-
gance. If the physicians of the century past tended to be humble and
conscientious, it was a good thing, since there was little accountability. If something went wrong, there were few consequences beyond
the loss of the patient. Today, as we all know, that's changed. Patients demand accountability and our legal system backs them up.
Yet incredibly, some doctors still don't get it. I remember a new
patient of mine, Joanna, who came in for an initial consultation. She
was a 39-year-old mother and had learned from the Internet about
the potential toxicity of mercury silver fillings in her mouth. She
was very concerned about the cavities that needed to be fixed and
those that were already filled with mercury. She went to see her
dentist and asked him what he knew about mercury being a dangerous material. He laughed at her. He said they were absolutely safe,
absolutely stable in the mouth. Then she asked him how he knew
they were safe. He had no answer.

Compounding these factors is something that's as true of medicine today as it was in the time of Dr. Miller and Dr. Wishnofsky or,
for that matter, the Middle Ages: medicine is highly conservative.
There have always been practitioners who refuse to change their
methods because that is how they've always practiced, that's what
they learned in medical or dental school. This is not entirely their
fault. The way our medical and dental schools teach their students is
for the most part "cookbook" style: look up the recipe; there's only
one correct way to diagnose and treat a patient. This approach leaves

little room for creative thinking, even though treating all medical cases in a similar "logical" order will result in a good percentage of them not responding well. And if they aren't improving, many clinicians have difficulty finding alternate reasons for the disorder.

Indeed, it's difficult to think outside the box. You know in your own life how we get into ruts. Knowing what to expect is comforting in many ways. When circumstances require a major change, the result is often stress. Even when a network changes the time it airs our favorite television show that may cause disruption and confusion. Changing jobs or partners can be terrifying. The fear of the unknown and fear of successfully living through the change is emotionally and physically taxing even if it means our lives will be happier and improved.

It's a fact, however, that many highly successful people embrace and even enjoy change. These mavericks have helped move our civilization forward for centuries. Without them we might still be in caves. Medicine too, like the proverbial turtle, can only make progress if it sticks its neck out. The best doctors in any era stick their necks out every once in a while to try innovative procedures. Although these new procedures must of course have demonstrated merit and some objective indication that they would be safe and effective alternatives to what the majority of practitioners are currently doing. Doctors who try them are the agents by which medicine has advanced over the years. We need these doctors to continue sound, safe medical and dental healthcare if we're going to enjoy future improvements in these fields. Yet as we've seen, such efforts are often resisted. Change is hard.

Not all change has taken place *within* the medical profession. Over the last 20 to 30 years patients have been lulled into a false sense of security. Reminded every day by the media and pharmaceutical companies of the advances and discoveries in medicine and dentistry, we tend to think that *any* medical or dental problem can be solved. And of course we're terribly busy. We tend to avoid or postpone visits to the doctor because we know that if something un-expected happens "they" will be able to fix it. Our work schedule is more important and takes all our time. That trip to Disneyworld takes priority over treating those decayed teeth. We no longer seri-ously consider that we might die or be permanently hurt by any-thing short of cancer and maybe a massive heart attack. Whatever our problem is, health care can fix, cure it or control it for us with a prescription drug or a new procedure just developed.

Yet, in fact, obstacles to health are everywhere. The lack of time a doctor can spend with a patient is only one. In a for-profit medi-cal insurance regime, your financial situation may seriously affect your health care. Bad eating habits and unhealthy life styles are easy to attain—indeed, almost irresistible for many. And just as in every other profession, there are good and bad doctors. You, the patient, cannot usually tell one from the other until something serious oc-curs. This could happen immediately or take years to appear.

Given the changed world we live in, we can't afford the trusting attitudes of 50 or 100 years ago. We have to be aware that there are alternatives to many types of treatment and understand that what the dentist or physician tells us might or might not be the correct diag-nosis or the best course of action.

For all these reasons, and in view of the other circumstances I've described in this book, I, as a medical professional, urge you *to take control of your own health care.* Your only protection is to question any diagnosis and treatment (or non-treatment) you may not understand right from the beginning. If you're told something that doesn't sound plausible or logical to you, investigate further or get a second opinion confirming that this is the proper course. These days, you'll often see your doctor consulting the Internet while you're in the office. You do the same! Read some evidence-based studies for yourself. You aren't going to become a doctor by doing that, but you are going to understand better what treatments might help and what treatments might not.

THE SEARCH FOR A DENTAL PRACTICE

It was a busy Thursday, about 11 in the morning. I had more patients in my schedule than I should have. I don't like keeping patients waiting: they can become nervous sitting in the waiting room. But my staff was terrific and up to the challenge, and so far I was on time. That was when the telephone call came in.

I was finishing bonding a white resin filling in the upper left premolar of Nyugen, when I saw Nina, my office manager, standing in the doorway. She didn't look happy. I like to keep Nina happy. When she's happy, I'm usually happy.

"Be right with you," I said warily.

A few minutes later I was standing in the hall with Nina. "What's up?"

"Mrs. Chen is on the phone," she whispered. "Her daughter, Tina, was up all night in severe pain and her dentist was not helpful at all. Mrs. Chen wants your advice about what Tina can do. She's not looking for you to see her today. She just has no idea what to do."

But Nina knew exactly what I was going to say. Some dentists do their job and go home, with no extra effort to help anyone beyond what is necessary. My job is to help people who need help. For all my years in practice, if a patient or anyone called who was in pain, I've made sure to see them immediately or as soon as possible. I consider it a mandate of my profession to treat these people on an emergency basis, and either relieve their pain or refer them to someone who can.

"Tell her to have Tina come over immediately. She may have to wait a short time but we'll work her into the schedule."

Tina was in my dental chair by noon. She was 28 years old. She held her lower right jaw with her hand and was obviously in pain. It didn't look like she had had any sleep the previous night. After reviewing her past history I asked her about her current dentist.

"I've been going to him for two years," she said. "His office was on the list from my insurance company. He just did three fillings in my teeth three months ago. I called him this morning and told him about this pain. He said it sounded like I needed root canal treatment. He said not to come in to see him as he doesn't do root canal treatment. He gave me the name and phone number of some other dentist he said does root canal treatment."

She was almost in tears.

"I tried calling this dentist several times and only got a machine. I left messages and finally they called me back. They said they couldn't see me for two weeks! I couldn't wait that long, even on pain medication. I called my dentist back and he said he couldn't help me. He again said to call the root canal dentist."

She looked at me and her face was fraught with fear.

"I didn't know what to do so I called my mother and she called you, her dentist."

I hear stories like this every few weeks. It's bad enough some dentists won't immediately see a person in pain who calls their office, but imagine refusing to see their own patient in times of real need.

"Let's take a look and a couple of x-rays. If I can, I'll get you out of pain today.

As it turned out, Tina had an acute alveolar abscess in her lower right molar. This is what people typically think of when they envision a toothache with swelling and pain. This situation was worse, however, because there *was* no swelling. The infection was in the mandibular jaw bone, causing pressure and pain. If not treated immediately, Tina would probably wind in a hospital emergency room within a day or two. Left untreated that long, she might have developed cellulitis, a serious diffuse bone infection, or perhaps bone necrosis.

After giving her local anesthesia, I drilled open the offending tooth. When the pulp of the tooth (where the nerve tissue resides) gets infected from the bacteria in the tooth decay, the pulp dies and necroses, that is, becomes gangrenous. The decay gases that build up inside the tooth have no where to go except out the bottom of the tooth (the root) and into the jawbone. By opening the top of the tooth, I released the pressure and allow the abscess to drain out of the tooth.

Within one day Tina's pain had subsided and the antibiotics I had given her had started to work. Mrs. Chen called later to thank me for seeing her daughter.

ↄ⟫

I hope this story illustrates how important it is to pick the right dental practice, regardless of the types of emergency. Tina should have known what her dentist's office protocols were for emergencies. In the United States, one trip to an emergency room can wipe out any savings an individual expects to gain from choosing a doctor just because he participates in a dental insurance plan. And consider the following before we consider the grave threats to health that neglected dental emergencies can pose.

There are good and bad dentists. Ironically, from the dentist's point of view, being a responsible, quality-oriented practitioner actually has many practical advantages. Tina became a patient of mine after that incident. She's sent me a dozen patients over the years. Whatever considerations kept her former dentist from helping her, they cost *him* money.

There are many reasons for choosing one dentist over another. Here are a few common ones:

♦ Your dentist is not only good looking, but single.

♦ Your dentist has a sexy foreign accent and a wonderfully throaty voice.

♦ Your dentist is your friend.

♦ Your dentist is your spouse's friend.

♦ Your dentist's office is right around the corner from where you work.

- ◆ Your dentist participates in your insurance plan.
- ◆ Your dentist's fees are, er, less costly than most.
- ◆ You've got a discount coupon.

I'm confident that you, dear reader, would never choose a dentist for any of these reasons. You probably don't make your living by betting at roulette, either, and dental roulette is asking for trouble since, in all aspects of business including healthcare, there are the good and the bad and the ugly. There is no way to know which is which by considering only one factor. Any type can charge high fees or low fees. Any type of dentist can have a great personality but so what? You in your capacity as patient are not dating them.

And you as a layperson have little chance of picking a good dentist out of the blue. To take control of your own health care, your must do your homework, You must evaluate as many aspects of the potential dental practice as you can before becoming a patient.

> How much is good dentistry worth to you?…Cheap or poor dentistry will cost you more in the long run.

⟪☙⟫

I left the office at lunchtime one day to make a deposit at my local bank. I had been to this bank hundreds of times over the years and simply used the drive-up teller lane. As I pulled up in the first lane, I saw the teller who usually assisted me behind the glass. She was an attractive 45ish woman, well dressed, moderately made-up, hair fashionably styled. She had always been friendly and always greeted me with a smile and a "Hello Dr. Robbins" at each visit.

This time was different.

"Hi Dr. Robbins." She wasn't smiling. "You're not my most favorite person today!"

I was caught off guard. All I could say was, "What's the matter?"

"I just returned from my dentist's office." she replied, "I had to go in as an emergency because his cap had fallen off again. My face is all numb."

The reader will note that this woman referred to another dentist, a dentist unknown to me, yet saw dentists as a homogeneous professional substance. *"All dentists are the same."* That's why I wasn't her favorite person that day. Yet this *was* a story I had heard over and over from new patients I saw on an emergency basis.

"This wasn't the first time this happened?" I asked, keeping a wary eye on the car behind me. Dental consultations are usually not conducted in the drive-in teller lane.

"Oh no. It's happened two other times since he made the cap last year."

"I see." Tact, I kept telling myself, is part of a good dentist's professional package. "You say it keeps falling off and you keep going back for him to put it back on?"

"That's right. Three times now."

"Right. Now, um, why do you return to him if it keeps falling off?"

The answer was predictable.

"Why?" She shook her head at my naïveté. "Because he doesn't charge me to put it back on!"

No matter how often people whom I meet socially or casually tell me stories like this, I'm astounded. You have no idea how many patients keep returning to the same dentist as their fillings continue to fall out or they still can't floss a new filling or they struggle with some other poorly done treatment that gets no better after returns to the dentist. Because they continue to pursue a failing treatment, I ask these people a hypothetical question. If you needed a heart transplant and after the surgery you looked like one of those little blue cartoon Smurfs, would you go back to the *same* heart surgeon to redo the failed transplant? You'd see immediately that something was terribly wrong. How many times would you go back to a car repairman if the same breakdown kept happening? Wouldn't you look for another serviceman who could repair the car correctly?

How much is good dentistry worth to you? Going back to a bad dentist several times for the same problem is not a good idea. If he could not fabricate a good crown originally, one that should last 10 to 20 years, why go back? It won't get any better. Cheap or poor dentistry will cost you more in the long run. Folks who hope to save money by having cheap dentistry the first time may think they're biding their time and can have the better procedure done later. Unfortunately that is not usually what happens. By the time the tooth or teeth need to be redone, sometimes only a couple of years later, there's too much damage and either it costs several times more than originally quoted or the bad teeth may have to be extracted. You might as well know the truth: bad dentistry can ruin your mouth permanently.

THE GOOD

A Website

Dentists who have modern progressive practices like prospective patients to know what they can offer. They are proud of their practices and many have their own websites. These sites can be loaded with useful information. The credentials of the dentist and sometimes the staff may be listed. The continuing education or resumé of the dentist may be listed, as may some of the more recent conferences or courses the dentist and staff attended. Pictures of the office are important, but look past the pretty waiting room furniture and see the treatment room equipment if it's shown. Can you see new technology and equipment? What does the site say about what diagnostic and treatment procedures the dentist uses? What kind of restorative options and materials are available? Do they offer nitrous oxide and is that important to you? Is there a dental hygienist to take care of your checkup needs, or does the dentist perform the dental checkups? Does the website give you other information that may be helpful for your own knowledge? Does it explain procedures and techniques they use and why they are good or better than others? Are there any testimonials from patients? Discount testimonials that only give a first name or initials. Anyone can make up those statements. If a patient is sincerely grateful and pleased by the treatment they received in the office, they should be willing to let the office use their full name. Lastly, is there a "Contact Us" page so that you can e-mail the office any questions or have someone at the office call you? Is there a name of a front desk person or administrator whom you can call and ask for by name? Do they offer to send office and practice information to you by mail or Internet if you request it?

A Curriculum Vitae

If your dentist offers a complete curriculum vitae, this is a great help. Has he or she attended many continuing-education seminars and conferences in the last few years? Remember that dental theory is evolving faster than many practices: post-graduate courses dentists might have attended six years ago are not as important as those taken recently: if dentists aren't constantly monitoring the dental field through periodicals and continuing education courses, they may be practicing in the past. And while you're at it, do reward extra points for any published peer-reviewed scientific journal articles or any lectures your prospective dentist may have given to other dentists. Articles printed in general-interest layperson magazines, on the other hand, don't tell you much.

What organizations does the dentist belong to, not counting the American Dental Association's affiliated groups and societies? In the United States, local county dental societies are almost always affiliated with the ADA. If you live in the States, does your dentist belong to the Academy of General Dentistry, a more independent national organization for general dentists only? How about membership in medical or toxicology organizations, or associations for specific dental procedures, such as the Academy of Cosmetic Dentistry, American Academy of Pain Management (TMJ or Facial pain conditions) or American Endodontic Society (devoted to root canal treatment)? The International Academy of Oral Medicine and Toxicology is especially progressive and provides their members with information about many new materials and techniques based on actual scientific evidence.

A Referral

An easy way to find a dental practice is by calling a dental specialist in your vicinity for a referral. Periodontists are specialists who treat gum disease and some may place surgical implants in addition to the usual periodontal care. As local patients filter through their offices, these specialists see a lot of dental work that has been performed in their area. They know who's good and who's not so good and can often provide you with two or three names of general dental practices they recognize as superior.

First Impression

How were you treated when you called the dental office for information or for an initial appointment? This "feeling" for an office is a valuable indicator. Does the person answering the telephone sound happy? Is she glad you called? Does she ask you what your concerns are and how the practice can help you? Does she answer your questions? Does she tell you about some of the services the office can offer?

If you make an appointment, do you get information and a confirmation in the mail? Is there a "welcome to the practice" letter enclosed?

John had visited another dental office immediately before switching to my practice. He'd called them to inquire about an appointment and was confronted immediately with a question.

"Do you have insurance?" the assistant asked, "and if so, what kind?"

Despite the rocky start, he set up an appointment with the hygienist for the following week.

When he arrived for his first visit, there were two staff members chatting at the front desk. He waited three or four minutes until one of them acknowledged him and gave him a questionnaire to fill out. There was no greeting. The office furniture was "from the stone age" and the waiting room was dark. Reading material of any interest was absent. The visit with the hygienist lasted 30 minutes and that included four x-rays. The dentist came in and spent less than five minutes examining John's mouth. The "cleaning" had taken all of 10 minutes and, when John ran his tongue around the inside of his mouth, he could tell his teeth were not totally clean.

He seemed embarrassed as he told me about this experience. I told him *I* was embarrassed because it reflected badly on my profession as a whole. He said he had learned his lesson and intended to be more careful in choosing a new dentist. He had gone to my website and called my office manager with questions about the practice. He said I had a great office staff and he felt good about his upcoming visit. He appreciated the welcome letter and practice information we sent to him after he made the appointment.

Why should it be otherwise?

Staff

If you prefer, stop in to see the office and meet the person you've talked to by telephone. Observing the activity and energy level of the office in person may help you decide if the practice is right for you. Is it confused and anxious? Is it laid back and calm? Is the waiting room comfortable emotionally? The last thing you want in a dental office is to be anxious. Do staff members seem to get along with one other or is there tension? Is there a lot of idle gossip and talking within earshot of the patients or is the tone a professional one?

How does the staff look? Do they have 15 earrings and a nose piercing? Are there tattoos exposed where you would prefer not to look? Remember, the appearance of the staff is a reflection of the dentist and his practice. Jewelry and slovenly attire on the clinical staff have no place in a professional office. Coordinated staff uniforms or scrubs are a nice touch. Is there hot coffee or tea, and cold water in the waiting room? Are the wall coverings older than dirt or is the waiting room upbeat and cheerful?

Does someone speak to you or come out into the waiting room to greet you as a new patient with a welcome or do they ignore you until you stand at the desk?

Do the office staff as well as the dentist attend continuing education courses? If they all take courses in their respective fields, you can assume dedication of the staff to the practice. It also suggests the desire and mission of the practice is to maintain a high standard of care for its patients.

Emergencies

What is the office protocol for emergency problems during non-office hours? Can the doctor be reached 24 hours a day through an answering service? Most offices now have pagers for the dentist that a patient can beep if an emergency occurs. Do you instead have to leave a message on an answering machine and hope that someone (hopefully, the dentist) will call in for messages frequently? Not a good option.

Does the dentist have another practice to cover his/her patients when away at a conference or on a vacation? Good dentists have to marvel that some doctors and dentists simply close their offices with no set, dependable referral for any of their patients who might have an emergency. It doesn't matter if it's for the day and the office re-opens the next morning or for a week's vacation. Being a doctor brings serious responsibilities for insuring the well-being of your patients. In most jurisdictions the doctor is only legally responsible for his or her own patients of record (patients that have been to the doctor's office recently), but inherent in the doctor's degree is a moral duty to help others as well.

⸙

My pager went off a Saturday morning in November while I was eating breakfast. I called back the number that was flashing in the pager display and reached a woman who sounded very stressed.

"Hello, Dr. Robbins. I'm sorry to bother you on a Saturday but I'm in trouble. I'm not one of your patients but I was hoping you could help me."

Patients often forget to give their name when I call them back. They expect me to know who they are from their telephone number and voice, and go right into describing their problem. This voice sounded sincerely apologetic. Most patients do feel guilty about bothering a doctor when their office is not open. But in my experience, although those who actually page doctors at off-hours rarely have problems serious enough to be seen immediately, those who do have serious, acute conditions do not contact doctors soon enough.

"To whom am I speaking?"

"Oh, sorry. My name is Eleanor Russell. My dentist apparently is away for the week and he just worked on a lower molar on Thursday. I tried calling his office and only got an answering machine. It said he was away at a meeting and if you have a dental emergency to call this other dentist. I tried that number also but got no answer since last night."

She was still apologizing. I appreciated her genuine

nervousness about calling a dentist on his day off, even though she wasn't my patient.

"Tell me what your problem is" I said.

"Since Thursday night I've been in pain. He told me I might need a root canal treatment on this tooth. I woke up this morning and have a swelling in my right cheek, down under the jawbone. I don't know if this can wait another week until he gets back. What do you think?"

I learned very early in my dental career that if you listen to a patient long enough, they will give you the diagnosis themselves. It was not the pain that concerned me. I can always get pain medication to a patient through their local pharmacy. But when she talked about a bad tooth and swelling overnight—*that* was a true emergency. Swelling under the jaw can quickly progress and start to block the airway. That's in addition to the infection and purulent accumulation in the tissues.

"Are you now taking any antibiotics?"

If she was on an antibiotic, the infection was pretty aggressive to be that swollen overnight. On the other hand, the infection might not be responding to the particular antibiotic prescribed.

"No, he said to call him if I had a problem."

"I need to see you as soon as possible in my office. You have a severe infection that needs attention today. Do you know where my office is located?"

We agreed to meet in three hours in my office.

When Eleanor arrived in my office, I greeted her over her apologies for bringing me out on a Saturday afternoon. She was an extremely pleasant 62-year-old black woman who may have weighed 300 pounds. I told her this was a real emergency and I knew she had to be seen.

I reviewed her medical history. She was on over a dozen medications for high blood pressure, diabetes, acid-reflux, cholesterol and others. When I was satisfied I could proceed— we always take blood pressure readings on patients reporting health problems—I examined her neck, face, mouth and teeth. I took an x-ray of a lower right molar that had a temporary filling in the top. This was the offending tooth. I could not even touch the tooth without her jumping. The temporary filling appeared to be pushing into the pulp of the tooth on the x-ray. There was visual evidence at the tip of the roots of an acute dental abscess—an infection.

"Eleanor, I am glad you came in today. You have a severe tooth abscess, and the infection and pus is spreading down your neck. I need to put you on a strong antibiotic. While you are here I'm going to give you Novocain and open the tooth so it can drain."

She was filled with apprehension. I talked with her a few more minutes and proceeded to treat the infection. She actually felt very little pain and I was done in 10 minutes. She got up and we went to the front desk. I gave her a prescription for an antibiotic and instructions for the following couple of days and told her to call me if things got worse.

"Eleanor, if you hadn't come in today, you'd have been in the hospital emergency room by tomorrow. I think you'll be all right now. Just follow the directions I gave you."

"I can't thank you enough for seeing me today." Her gratitude was clear. "I want to set up an appointment for you to do the root canal treatment. My dentist doesn't do them and would have sent me somewhere else anyway. I think I am going to change dentists to you, if it's all right?"

"I appreciate the vote of confidence. If you can call Monday morning and ask Nina for an appointment, we should do that root canal treatment this week. It was nice meeting you."

I knew when she left she'd be comfortable and pain-free within 24 hours but I always call emergency patients later the same day just to make sure and in case they have any questions. It also makes it less likely I'll be paged again that day.

People such as Eleanor demonstrate how genuinely most patients appreciate efforts made to help them. She's been a patient in my practice for over six years now and has sent me quite a few of her friends as patients.

The bottom line: guidelines for dental emergency calls during non-office hours are important. Make sure when you check out dental practices you know exactly what their policy is when the doctor is away. There are several ways doctors can responsibly handle emergency calls when their office is normally closed.

Telephone

Answering Service. This was the most common method for many years. When a patient calls they actually get a real live person answering the call. These operators triage the call to determine how serious or important it is and then either notify the doctor or keep the message until the next day the office is open. Originally (and still for some practices) the operator actually telephoned the doctors and gave them the message over the phone. More frequently, operators now relay the message to a doctor's cell phone or pager. The message can be a tone or, in the case of personal digital assistants (PDAs such as Treo® or Palm®), operators can relay a written message that appears on the doctor's portable view screen.

From the patient's point of view this is the best and fastest method of reaching the doctor. But it is the *doctor's* responsibility to assure that his answering service knows how to reach him. If he switches off the device, if he is out of range of cell towers or out of the country, he simply cannot be reached.

Answering Machine. Many offices now use a telephone answering machine combined with a relay service. The patient calls and gets an answering machine message. The office then follows one of two procedures. Either the machine's message asks the patient to leave a voice message and their telephone number so that the doctor can call them back, or callers may leave a message on the machine, but receive an additional option to call a second telephone number and punch in their own telephone. This second service relays the patient's callback number to a pager or cell phone carried by the doctor. He gets the number and returns the call.

From the patient's point of view, the first option can be a problem. The return call could come in minutes or at the end of the day. The system requires first that doctor or someone from the office call in to retrieve the messages. This is a very bad system for someone with an emergency. The second system allows the patient to get their phone number directly to the doctor. In both cases, however, it's the doctor's responsibility to get the messages and return the call.

Direct telephone line. Some practices have an answering machine (or a telephone number that appears on office cards, bills and documents) that provide patients with a telephone number they can call and directly reach the doctor. This might be another office location, a clinic where the doctor works, or a cell phone the doctor carries. This is clearly the best option for a patient who wants to reach a doctor immediately but is rarely available for the obvious reasons that it is open to abuse.

Breadth of Services

It's wise to determine beforehand what procedures a prospective dental practice performs beyond general dental practice. You may want a practice that treats most root canal teeth without referral to an outside dentist. Would you want some periodontal procedures (beyond scaling and polishing during routine checkups) performed in the same office? Will the dentist treat your eight-year-old without referring her to a specialist? Is that important to you? Find out.

Modern Equipment and Technology

While state-of-the-art equipment is no guarantee that a dentist will be a superior surgeon, having little or no modern equipment does prevent a dentist from being a superior one. It is not just the "whistles-and-bells" of technology that makes it appear as a superior dental practice. The latest equipment allows the dentist to be more accurate in the diagnosis and treatment of dental problems. Don't be afraid to ask the prospective dentist's representative what technologies the dentist is using. Here are some examples of new equipment:

High-efficiency mercury air cleaners remove mercury vapors released when an amalgam filling is drilled out of a tooth. Use of these devices is only one of a range of protocols that must be followed to safely remove these silver-colored fillings from patients' mouths. The IQAir Dental Mercury air cleaners are the best and most efficient I have found.

High speed electric handpieces are smoother and stronger while drilling and make very little noise. They require less force on the tooth and therefore allow for greater accuracy.

Newer dental materials for the restoration of decayed teeth, materials that incorporate nanotechnology and bonded hybrid-composite resins, both last longer and cause less postoperative sensitivity and fewer overall problems than older materials. Avoid offices using metal in crowns unless these crowns are made of 100% pure gold, that is, gold or gold and platinum.

Intra-oral dental cameras have probes that can be placed over a tooth in the mouth for magnified photos. The images show cracks and breakdown of teeth that may not be visible by the examining dentist while looking in the dental mirror. These images are often essential for getting insurance companies to pay claims.

Computer monitors and educational programs in each dental operatory allow the patient to actually see their teeth or gums on the screen. Patients can better understand what is wrong and why recommended procedures must be performed. The patient can see, for instance, the actual breakdown of teeth due to old amalgam mercury fillings. A dentist can show instructional and educational programs on the monitors so patients know what to expect from a recommended treatment.

Digital dental radiology or digital x-rays reduce radiation exposure. Although the dentist can manipulate the image to better see various parts of the teeth, there are limitations. These images are more expensive to take and many offices charge more. The sensor is not very flexible and placing it in the mouth is difficult and painful in a large proportion of cases; positioning it for certain tooth views is sometimes impossible. There is still controversy between dentists who swear that digital x-rays are the best and those that do not see enough difference to justify the huge cost to install the digital equipment and the commensurate charge to the patient. My personal experience suggests that x-rays are more easily taken and read using traditional x-ray film and that digital radiographs are not quite as good yet.

Laser technology has revolutionized surgical correction and removal of soft tissue in the mouth and surrounding tissues. Although most lasers have not been generally approved for cutting tooth structure, they have proven far superior to other technologies for surgery on gingiva, mucosa, connective tissues, palatal tissues and other soft tissues in the mouth. No bleeding and little post-operative pain are major advantages. The few lasers that are approved for cutting tooth structure for restorations are fast becoming serious competitors to the traditional dental drills. Again high cost to install and increased cost to the patient remain stumbling blocks to widespread acceptance.

Non–fluoridated toothpastes and polishing pastes are the way to go today. Fluoride is not as effective as we've thought for over 50 years and the newer "remineralizing" toothpastes do far more to protect your teeth and health. A dentist who carries these products is really on the ball and up-to-date with current scientific evidence and technology. These newer toothpastes are unfortunately available only on a dentist's prescription.

Toxin Protocols

Nutritional Protocols. More and more dental offices are offering nutritional counseling for their patients. We review the supplements patients are taking and advise them about basic nutritional and nutraceutical (vitamins, minerals and supplements) adjustments or additions that might be helpful for their physical and mental health and protection. I consider supplements used when removing mercury from the teeth as part of this nutritional counseling. We want a strong healthy patient to increase the probability that removal of the toxic mercury and exposure to any mercury vapor will not seriously affect their health. If a dental office offers this service, this shows concern about the overall patient's condition, not just their mouth. It also indicates the dentist has attended more advanced continuing education since they graduated dental school, because these subjects are not taught in any detail in their training.

Mercury Protocols. Biological dentistry emphasizes the "first do no harm" creed of the medical profession. Using *any* material or instrument in the mouth or body that is not biocompatible with human physiology is prohibited. When I look into a patient's mouth and see anything that does not comply with this fundamental principle, I recommend the patient have it removed and/or replaced. A dentist's attitude towards mercury should be one of your most compelling signs of a progressive practice.

Fluoride Protocols. Biological dentistry mandates that any chemical, compound or agent used in a patient's mouth be biocompatible with the patient's health. It is the dentist's responsibility to promote the health of the whole patient, not just "fix a tooth." Dentists are not repairmen and if a dentist practices like a repairman, that is not the dentist you want. Use of a toxic material which has limited, questionable benefits for the mouth, while harming the patient's overall physiology is forbidden. Ask your prospective dental practice about their protocols for use or non-use of fluoride for children and adults. I recommend not choosing a practice that still recommends for children any topical fluoride treatment or fluoride-containing product.

Metals Used in Treatment. As we've seen, many metals used in crowns are not biocompatible with your body, can be harmful to tissues in the mouth or can accumulate in your body. Ask your dentist specifically what percentage of the different metals used are in the crowns the dentist makes. You will find the answer helpful.

Participating Insurance Plans

Whether or not a dentist office participates in various insurance plans is not an accurate measure of their quality of dental care. However, participating in insurance plans *can* be an indicator of poor quality. Many offices belong to a couple of dental plans. If a dental office participates in many dental plans (perhaps six or more), be prepared for a pace in the office that is geared to profit generated by volume. A quality dental practice earns respect and profits through what it does, not how many it does it to.

How a Dental Maintenance Organization (DMO) Works

In the US, a dental office may participate in a dental health maintenance organization (DMO), which is the dental equivalent of a medical HMO. Such an arrangement does not allow the dentist to practice high quality dental care. Such practices must perforce operate as "Grand Central Stations," moving patients in and out as quickly as possible.

A DMO-participating practice is paid a very small amount each month for each DMO-covered patient that chooses to enroll in that specific office. This can be as low as $4 or $5 per patient per month. For that $50 per year, the dentist is usually required to perform all basic dental procedures including checkups, x-rays, extractions and fillings without additional fees or compensation. On the other hand, the dentist is paid this *whether the patient comes into the office or not.* The dentist must also perform major dental work like crowns and dentures at a very low contracted fee (maybe 5% or 10% of their regular fee). There is clearly the potential here for major abuses of normal dental standards of care.

♦ The dental office makes more money if the patient *doesn't come in for an appointment*. They get paid anyway.

♦ The faster the patients are treated the more patients can be seen in a short period of time. Minimal or incomplete treatment simply pays better.

♦ If a filling or crown, for example, is not done, the office makes more money, since the dentist is paid no more for performing that procedure than if he or she did *not*. Needed work may be overlooked or avoided.

♦ Fast dental treatment leads to sloppy dental treatment and problems, pain or retreatment afterwards.

♦ Buying the cheapest materials and equipment or using an inexpensive dental laboratory to fabricate crowns and dentures, saves the dentist money, but leads to early failure of any dental work. Every time a tooth is retreated, less tooth structure remains. This means that deeper and bigger holes progress in teeth with more root canal treatments and extractions needed. Ultimately the patient pays more for frequent treatment on the same teeth.

When I belonged to Aetna/US Healthcare DMO many years ago, I kept the same high quality of dental care for all my patients. I began to lose income treating the DMO-covered patients because I was not paid for the time it took to diagnose and treat them properly. On top of that Aetna was cheating me out of thousands of dollars each year by not entering my submitted procedures correctly each month. As of this date I still have a lawsuit pending against Aetna/US Healthcare for their deceptive business practices—racketeering in my opinion—and cheating me out of reimbursement from the 1990s.

You may find the fees in a quality practice slightly higher and your out-of-pocket costs more, but the service will usually be far superior to a quickie insurance or DMO-based dental office. Future dental problems will be minimal because time was taken performing the dental treatment as well.

Last Word on the Good

In a good dental practice, the dentist will have a long initial consultation with you if you have several teeth that need treatment. A short consultation can be adequate if, for example, there are only a couple of teeth that need small fillings. However if there's a lot of work to be done, your dentist should outline several critical issues:

♦ What's wrong in your mouth (gum disease, decay, missing teeth, bite problems, defective restorations, etc.)

♦ What will happen if nothing is treated

♦ The dentist's recommended best treatment for your case

♦ Any alternative treatments to the best treatment

♦ Possible additional complications that may occur, causing the need for further treatment

♦ The time and appointments needed to accomplish the planned treatment

♦ The estimated fees for the recommended treatment and an indication of what additional costs might accrue if things don't go as planned.

Once the consultation is complete, other members of the dental staff can help with questions about appointments, payment and payment plans, insurance, etc. You must feel comfortable with the whole office—dentist and staff—to have a successful dental experience.

Occasionally, a treatment may not go as expected, no matter how good your dentist. Unexpected results are common in any medical or

> Quality treatment = less treatment and pain = dental health = overall body health

dental treatment. But it's *how* the doctor handles the problem that determines the quality of a practice. If your dentist fills the bill I've described in this section, you can expect to be treated properly even where things don't go as you both hoped.

If you need advanced treatment, that is, more than a couple of fillings, expect a complete consultation with the dentist. Expect to be told and understand all the proposed treatment and fees—before treatment begins. If your dentist starts treating you without explanation or telling you what the fee will be, start looking for another dental practice.

THE BAD AND THE UGLY: SIGNS

As important as it is to know how to locate a good, high-quality dental practice, it's equally important to know when to *leave* a dental practice. One of the biggest mistakes patients make is waiting too long to question treatment when a dental event occurs that does not seem like a common problem.

When you're in the wrong hands, there are usually warning signs that suggest the dental care you are getting is unacceptable or downright bad.

✆

Mohammed was shaking my hand very vigorously. He was smiling and looking from me to my hygienist and back again to me.

"Thank you very much, Dr. Robbins. That was the best tooth cleaning I've ever had. It didn't hurt and my teeth feel much cleaner now."

He was clearly impressed. Actually his mouth was not bad. He just had tons of calculus around the teeth and under the gums.

"I was surprised you had so much tartar under your gums Mohammed. You told me you just saw your old dentist last year. Didn't they get the tartar out like we did?"

I already knew the answer. Many patients don't know how a scaling and polishing should be done. They are given a very fast once-over and set up for a six-month recall. This is especially true for patients from overseas. Dental care in third world countries is usually not a pleasant or rewarding experience. We're seeing more and more "foreign" patients as local companies hire them for special employment needs. Their dental health knowledge is minimal and they don't expect much. Most are pleasantly surprised at how complete our office treated them.

Mohammed thought a moment. "My dentist only looked in my mouth for a quick minute when I had an appointment. He then did my tooth cleaning himself, but it only took a few minutes and then he was done. My teeth never felt or looked the way they do now!"

He went to my front desk and made appointments for his whole family.

The Speedy Check-up

The speedy check-up is a very bad sign. The dentist takes only two or three minutes to examine your mouth. Alternatively, the speedy dentist doesn't examine you at all; the dental hygienist is the only one who examines you. But who then is checking for decay and cavities? Who is looking at and diagnosing the x-rays? Who is looking for changes in the soft tissue in your mouth that may be evidence of cancer or some other pathology?

The Speedy Cleaning

Your dental scaling and polishing takes only five minutes. Wow. The teeth of even the best brusher and flosser usually require more than a few minutes. Is the hygienist (or dentist if there is no hygienist) flossing your teeth after they are polished? Do you still have brown or dark stain on your teeth after the cleaning? Do your gums bleed when you floss and has someone in the office talked to you about why they bleed? Do they explain gum disease and show you how to floss and brush more effectively? (See Figure 4-1, p. 218.)

Periodontal Chart? What Periodontal Chart?

Periodontal charting is the annual measurement and recording of gum pockets around your teeth. The conscientious dentist (or hygienist) systematically probes around each tooth to see if the sulcus (the crevice between tooth and gum) is too deep. Periodontal charting also shows the level of gum and gum recession around the teeth. Deep pocketing is usually a sign of gum disease and must be treated early to avoid serious problems—tooth loss, loose teeth, an ugly smile due to gum recession, root decay—at a later time. These measurements should be taken at least once a year and if your dentist's office isn't doing it, something's wrong. (See Figures 4-2 and 4-3.)

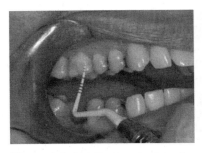 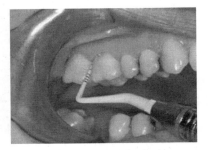

Figure 4-2 & 4-3: A periodontal probe is used to measure gingival sulcular depth (pockets) to gauge evidence of periodontal disease. This information is recorded in the periodontal chart.

But Grandma, What a Big Tooth You Have!

A Chicklet, for the younger among my readers, is a once-popular brand of gum. Chicklets came as rectangular pieces of gum, uniformly bright white, with rounded fronts and backs. If your new tooth restoration looks like a Chicklet—huge and with no fine detail

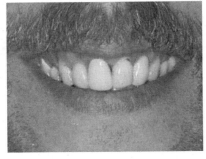

Figure 4-4. Crown too big.

compared to the look of the other teeth in your mouth—you're in trouble. (See Figure 4-4.) Except in special cases, a restoration should accurately replace the size and shape of a normal tooth in that location. If it feels or looks much bigger than your natural tooth, it can cause problems later on, problems that are irreversible. Gum disease or tooth decay from an ill-fitting crown, or tooth movement causing crossing of teeth and/or cosmetic problems are all potential consequences of a poorly shaped tooth restoration.

Uneasy Rests the Crown

If you have to return over three times before a new crown or laboratory restoration can be fitted to the tooth, something's wrong. A well-drilled, well-prepared tooth and a good impression technique are both standards for a good dentist. The dental laboratory can make a restoration for your tooth that will usually fit the first time unless:

♦ The dentist prepared the tooth incorrectly or badly.

♦ The dentist took a bad impression and sent it to the lab anyway.

♦ The dental laboratory is a quick, cheap lab doing below-average work.

No Room to Floss

If you cannot floss a tooth after it was repaired or restored, you've got a serious problem. If you cannot floss, food becomes impacted, plaque and bacteria accumulate between the teeth and under the gum. This causes bleeding and sometimes pain. If left to continue, your gums will recede permanently and your supporting bone be permanently destroyed. Decay will quickly get into the tooth causing failure of the restoration. On a front tooth, the result will be a cosmetic nightmare as illustrated in Figure 4-5, page 218.

When Fillings Fall

Does the white filling or crown you just had inserted keep falling out? It doesn't matter if the dentist puts it back in or places a new one, and it doesn't matter if he doesn't charge you. What matters is that it was *made wrong*. A proper filling or crown will not fall out.

> If your dentist tells you *not* to floss a tooth, *change dentists*.

What about this? A tooth restoration, made by a dental laboratory, keeps falling out *years* after it was completed, even though the dentist tries to re-cement it each time. Actually, this is a different situation from the first. All laboratory-made tooth restorations will eventually fail. They might decay underneath or the materials might wear out, break or crack as a result of long-term use. Sometimes the dentist may be able to clean out the tooth and replace (re-cement or rebond) the restoration in the tooth. However, if the crown or onlay falls out more that twice in a short time—a month perhaps—it should not be reused and a new one should be made. If the faulty work is not replaced, decay will quickly attack the tooth underneath and eventually require a larger restoration, root canal treatment or an extraction if the tooth is severely decayed. Your laboratory-made restorations should last 10 to 20 years with normal use. If your dentist keeps putting the same final restoration—crown, veneer or onlay—back in your tooth without telling you a new one is needed, *change dentists*.

Strange Cases of Emerging Metal

You've just had a *new* porcelain crown fitted and you look in your mouth and you can see metal on the chewing surface.

Hey, the whole point of making a metal crown with a porcelain covering is *for cosmetics*. If the crown has dark metal showing through the top surface, the crown must be returned to the dental laboratory to be remade with a new (and attractive) porcelain covering. However the tooth might have to be drilled *again* and a new impression taken. This is *not* good dentistry.

In some cases it may be necessary to deliberately fit a crown with a metal top. If this *is* the case, the dentist should alert you *in advance.*

Wear of the porcelain or plastic coatings of metal crowns is of course inevitable, but takes place over five to eight or more years.

A worse version of this sort of mistake is when the dentist does not calculate the correct thickness needed for the porcelain crown. When this crown is finally put on the tooth, the dentist drills patches of the porcelain away for the bite to fit. (See Figure 4-6.) Or the dentist leaves the porcelain covering so thin that it soon begins to chip away (as in the Figures 4-7 and 4-8, p. 218). Rotten teeth are bad enough. Why do people put up with rotten dentistry?

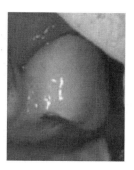

Figure 4-6: This new crown needed excessive bite adjustment due to poor construction.

DENTISTS AND PHYSICIANS: A COMPARISON OF SPECIES

For all their apparent similarities, dentists and physicians are two different animals.

In medical school, physicians are taught to work together for the benefit of the patient's health. Referrals are common from one doctor to another, even within their same specialty, because the other doctor might have more experience with a particular condition. Physicians work together in hospitals and clinics. They are more extroverted and seem to have more communication skills, though most are not great communicators anyway. Many physicians and specialists have joined forces and have formed groups in which they practice and cross-cover during down time. Nowadays they are taught to consider many alternative treatments for a medical problem. There is more than one way to support the health of a patient.

Dentists on the other hand are basically introverts. Many have ego issues and have trouble referring a patient to another dentist. They've got the idea that there's something wrong with themselves if they're not able to treat the patient's dental problem themselves. Referring the patient to another dentist is a sign of defeat for these dentists.

I'm among those dentists who are trying to reverse this tendency. I encourage my patients to be skeptical of what I say and recommend to them. I ask them to investigate the situation themselves either on the Internet or by obtaining a second opinion from another dentist. My patients appreciate the openness to discuss other possibilities for their health care.

◖◗

Barbara was a 48-year-old woman who appeared depressed to be in my office and in my dental chair. She was a statistician for an insurance company and so was analytical by nature. She started the conversation.

"Dr. Robbins, I want you to know I have been going to the dentist religiously, every six months for over 25 years. My dentist, Dr. Swain, was great. Whenever I had an appointment we always discussed all sorts of things in our lives. He would check my mouth and fix whatever he recommended I needed to have fixed. So why is my mouth in such bad shape?" She was obviously frustrated. "I've had to have some teeth taken out because they were cracked. My fillings keep falling out and need to be replaced. I have such *bad teeth!*"

I've heard this type of complaint hundreds of times. Patients would do what the dentist told them to do and still have terrible decay or gum disease. Probing their gums would sometimes reveal moderate to advanced periodontal disease, with deep, bleeding pockets around some of the teeth and the commensurate bone loss and gum recession. I often discover that these patients had never been referred to a periodontist in the earlier stages. Usually by the time I saw them, the damage was severe enough to require some teeth to be extracted. The whole history would point to the previous dentist not wanting to "give up the patient" to another dentist or specialist or simply not knowing about or recognizing gum disease. It's hard to say which is worse: not knowing basic periodontal diagnosis and treatment or not getting the patient the best professional help available. However, none of this turned out to be Barbara's problem.

I had just examined her mouth and noted many crowns and some missing teeth. "Tell me what happened to that missing lower right molar," I asked.

She took a deep breath. "Well, about five years ago, Dr. Swain found yet another cavity under the silver filling in that lower right tooth. He said it was deep and needed root-canal treatment to save the tooth. I went through a terrible experience with the root-canal treatment even though he did it himself. He later put a filling in the tooth but that broke after a year and it needed a crown. I had the crown done but after a year I had pain again. Dr. Swain took an x-ray and told me the tooth had abscessed again. It needed some sort of surgery in the bone near the root. An oral surgeon did the surgery.

"It was never right after that and needed to be extracted last year. I paid thousands of dollars to save that tooth and now Dr. Swain is talking about drilling down two other teeth for a bridge. I thought I should get another opinion."

☙

Barbara was a smart person and it wasn't her fault that she didn't know much about dental procedures. But, it was too bad it took her so long to realize there was a problem and get a second opinion. She'd already had experiences with Dr. Swain with other fillings he placed that fell out repeatedly.

What were the warning signs that Barbara missed?

First. Assuming a patient is doing at least a minimum job brushing and flossing and seeing their dentist regularly for their checkups, scalings and polishings, a new filling should last seven to 20 years before needing replacement. Usually a white bonded resin filling fails because of decay in the remaining tooth. If it is a mercury silver filling, it usually fails because the filling itself corrodes, cracks the tooth and then breaks off or allows decay underneath. The fact that her fillings kept falling out soon after they were placed should have been a big red warning flag that the job was probably not performed well.

Second. Root canal treatment is almost always successful if performed properly. (Unfortunately some root canal techniques—barbaric, in my view—are prone to failure.) If successful, the tooth can be expected to last one's whole lifetime without a new root canal procedure. If the root-canal treatment fails within a short time—say, under two years—this is a possible red flag that something may not have been done properly. How does the patient know what has happened? The dentist should explain any difficulty he encountered while performing the treatment *at the time of the root-canal appointment*. If a root-canal treatment fails, the dentist was usually aware of a potential problem when he performed the procedure in the first place. He should have explained the difficulty to the patient at the time of the procedure so the patient understood the possibility of failure and could accept the consequences.

Third. If a dental filling breaks within a year, it was probably the wrong way to restore the tooth. The tooth probably needed a crown or onlay in the first place. A porcelain restoration would better protect the tooth from pain, decay and cracking. A simple, large filling cannot effectively do that because it flexes too much, cracking and causing pain.

Fourth. In Barbara's case, the tooth was extracted less than two years after it was crowned. Crowns used to restore teeth should last 10 to 20 years or more. In all likelihood, this tooth restoration was a failure because it was not evaluated properly. Alternatively, the procedure itself was not performed skillfully. If she didn't get a second opinion when her fillings started falling out, Barbara certainly needed a second opinion after the tooth re-abscessed.

Dentists and Dentists: Comparison Shopping

You need a decent sweater. Let's see, where should you go? Maybe just pop into the first place you pass. Or, wait a minute, maybe that store where they offer discount stuff. Actually, there's a lot of advertising for sweaters on the Internet and even in the newspapers. Hmm. Could always ask a couple of friends where *they* go.

So you pick a place, go in and compare their sweaters. You look at materials, colors, quality, fit and price. If the store employees are friendly and helpful, that encourages you to do business with them. If you like all those things you take it to the cash register to pay for it. The clerk enters the item and tells you the price. You either pay by cash, or charge it or use a check.

You take the sweater home and put it on just before going out for the evening. The sleeve tears at the shoulder. You're a bit disgusted. The next day, you dig out the receipt and take the thing back to the store for a refund. It wasn't your fault that the sweater was defective. The store representative accepts the sweater and asks you if you want a replacement sweater or a refund of your money. You take the dough and go to another store and look at other sweaters.

That's how a business transaction works.

Dental practices are businesses too, but they're businesses with a difference. The transaction chain begins the same way, though. You suddenly realize for some reason that you need a dentist.

Where do you find a dental practice? Going to the nearest dentist or going to a practice that offers a discount is obviously risky, especially given what you now know. You need to research local dental practices because this will decrease your chance of an unhappy and possible unhealthy experience. We've looked at some of the ways you can do this research.

As with choosing a clothing store, asking friends may be a good option. Remember though: all your friends go to *someone.* They can't all be great. So at least ask how long your friends have been going to the particular dental practice, how has the dental work held up and lasted and how does it look? Quality dental work should last many years without problems.

Once you find a practice that appears to offer the services you want, you become a patient. Your new dentist should tell you ahead of time what treatment needs to be performed—if any—and what the fees are. Once you've had that procedure performed and go all innocently to the front desk, there shouldn't be any surprises. If the planned treatment had to be changed by the dentist, he or she should have alerted you to that change—and the probable change of fee—before leaving the room.

Do you pay for the treatment immediately or does the dental office wait for your insurance payment before you pay anything? This is a business decision each office makes. Do you need a payment plan or an installment loan? Many offices now have immediate financing options you can use to pay for your treatment.

If you go home and have problems with the treatment, can you return to the office and get your money back? No, of course not. This is not a product, it's a service. It's the skill and knowledge of the dentist that determines the success of the procedures. However your dentist should see you *immediately* should a problem arise from any recent dental treatment.

This last point is why *investigating a dental practice before you become a patient is so very important.* You cannot "return" a dental procedure or undo a service if it doesn't work out. Dental care involves teeth and gum surgery—the drilling or cutting of tissue. Once the tooth is drilled or the gums are changed, there is no way to return things to their original state. If your tooth or mouth doesn't feel good or is no longer healthy or attractive, what good is a discount coupon, an insurance payment or a low fee? The damage has been done permanently. If you are fortunate, and even if the condition is bad, a quality dentist may be able to improve or repair the result to bring things to a more satisfying conclusion. But prevention of the problem is the best solution: find a quality dental practice at the beginning.

In many ways then, seeing to your dental needs is unlike buying a sweater. Yet as I said at the start of this section, *dentistry is also a business*. Dentists open and carry on in these businesses in order to make money. It's fair to say that most dentists, if they should come suddenly into, say, $10,000,000, would retire. So, since they're running businesses, we expect them to behave in a business-like way. They must be open in manner and attitude and welcome patients asking questions, just like retail merchants do. They must explain in detail all the services they recommend for the patient. How can the patient make an informed decision to continue treatment if they are not informed? It's elemental, isn't it? So why don't more dentists follow these simple business principles?

Problem #1: Many dentists have a difficult time simply talking to patients.

Problem #2: Many dentists don't listen to patients and learn what they really want.

Problem #3: Many dentists don't take time to explain the diagnosis and treatment options to patients.

Problem #4: Many dentists cannot talk fees to patients.

Problem #5: Some dental offices do not help patients with payments for their services.

Problem #6: Some dentists refuse to take responsibility for the bad dental care they provide.

Some of these problems can be solved if the dentist delegates duties to his staff members who are better communicators. But when it comes to dental treatment, the dentist must explain his findings directly to you. You should be given time if you need it to decide on what the final treatment will be. Do not blindly accept the first recommendation a dentist makes until you fully understand the pros and cons. You don't want a doctor with an ego problem that can interfere with effective communication with you. You want a doctor who will listen and explain your dental conditions and address your unique concerns over the procedures.

Again and again I urge you to remember: in most dental practices, patients are "buying" the dentist and, like all consumers, they must do their homework and control the decision-making process. How much is good dentistry worth to you? Cheap or poor dentistry will cost you more in the long run.

SOME FINAL CONSIDERATIONS

When I was 14 in Queens, New York, my junior high school class decided to stage a Saturday roller-skating party at a local skating rink. In that remote era, most 14-year-olds hadn't actually tackled the dating of a girl, so among the guys I knew, an event as promising as a roller-skating party quickly became the subject of half our conversations.

Two weeks before the event, I was in a doctor's office with my mother. Dr. Stine was an ear, nose and throat man and he was looking down my throat. I remember he wore a white jacket embroidered with his name in blue on the left side of the chest. He was wearing a headband with this gigantic round mirror that pivoted off the front to reflect an examination light next to me. He was looking into my mouth and he wasn't smiling.

"How long has he had the sore throat?" he asked my mom. In those days, a parent, usually a mom, always went into the examination room with the kid and the godlike doctor spoke to the parent, not the kid. For Dr. Stine, I was just a throat.

"About three weeks," she answered. "He's had three sore throats and infections over the last six months. He has trouble breathing because his tonsils get so big." As if on cue I wheezed a breath.

"Well, they're infected and enlarged." Dr. Stine gave the throat a final squint. "They're blocking about ¾ of his airway now. I can see pustules coming out of the lymph tissue itself." I had to silently consider how disgusting that must be.

Dr. Stine put down his mouth mirror and switched off the light. He sat back. "They have to come out. It should be done next week after he's been on antibiotics for a week to fight the infection and shrink the glands. It's a little tricky taking them out at his age but we can do the procedure right in the office here."

This was enough to make anyone nervous. The important question had to be asked. I cleared my throat with some difficulty.

"There's a skating party in two weeks," I said. Dr. Kline regarded me without expression. "Will I be able to go to the party the week after the surgery?"

It was as if a fly had just landed on the doctor's nose and he answered as easily as he might bat that fly away. "You'll be fine a few days after the surgery," he said, looking me straight in the eye for the first time. "You should make that party, no problem." He resumed his discussion of the surgery with my mother.

On the day of the surgery I was told I'd be awake during the procedure. They sat me in a chair, put my head back against a headrest and affixed a metal spring band around my wrist. I didn't know it at the time but this was the grounding connection for a hyfrecator, a primitive coagulating device that included a hand-held electrode the doctor would use to stop bleeding. Dr. Stine opened my mouth and injected my tonsils with anesthetic and without preamble. There was no, and I'm putting it mildly here, no hand holding or other expressions of concern for the torment that was about to be inflicted on me. Dr. Stine, in a convincing imitation of Jack Ketch the hangman, just got on with his grim business, which I guess he figured somebody had to do. He cut my tonsils out and burned the bleeding area. The smell was unbearable.

When it was over, Dr. Stine told my parents to keep me in bed for a few days. Although it would "probably be uncomfortable," they should try to give me cold foods and ice cream to help keep the swelling and pain down. Dr. Stine didn't prescribe any pain medication and sent me home with my parents.

I lost over seven pounds during the first five days. My throat was on fire and the pain was so bad, I couldn't eat or drink much of anything. After two days the surgery area hemorrhaged and I was rushed bleeding to the hospital emergency room. Dr. Stine applied his hyfrecator again and home I went. It was two weeks before the nightmare began to abate at all but, as you see, I survived.

Now, as we approach the end of this book, I must tell you, patient readers, that this experience exerted considerable influence on me and on my attitude towards doctors. What I remember most about what seriously bothered me during this first taste of surgery was not the pain and suffering I went through. It was that this doctor, this man we honored with our trust and respect because he was a doctor, this man had purposely lied to me and to my parents. He knew the post-surgical course was not going to be easy. He knew I wouldn't be able to eat anything and I would have trouble swallowing anything, even water. He knew I'd be in great pain. And he knew there was no way in hell I was going to any skating party.

Why did he lie?

I have to tell you, I've pondered that question for 40 years. He could have told us the truth so we were better prepared for what would inevitably follow. He could have given me pain medication to help me get through the first few days. He could have done many things. The terrible truth is inescapable: this cold-hearted clinician just didn't care.

I've written this book to give you support in your dealings with the branch of health care that I know and love, but you can apply its broader lessons to the wider field of medicine. I've written it to help you make the decisions you'll need to make. I've written it because many dentists, just like many people whatever their profession, are honest, caring, inquisitive and wise, but many other dentists, like many other people, are sly, indifferent, greedy or lazy. There are dentists who choose every day not to reveal the whole truth to a patient. There are dentists who are by nature insensitive and indifferent practitioners. There are dentists and doctors whose only real weakness is their weakness: they'd rather lie than tell you the truth about your condition, lest it make you unhappy and perhaps cause you not to like them.

"Murder will out," MacBeth mused, and by "murder" he meant the truth. It's one of the greatest achievements of our post-Enlightenment culture that the truth sooner or later displaces earlier "truths." And the tide of understanding that's beginning to sweep away the old "truths" of dentistry is no small thing. Everywhere on the planet, in the largest and the smallest countries, in the greatest cities and the smallest towns, dentists are fixing people's teeth. A revolution in this branch of medicine is a revolution indeed.

I wrote this book so you'll stand up and play your part in that revolution by having your questions answered honestly and directly. You're not alone any more and information is no longer in the possession of the few. Never let any dentist, doctor or health care provider talk down to you. You have a right to ask questions and be fully informed about your condition and treatment and any financial obligation this may entail.

How much is good dentistry worth to you? Cheap or poor dentistry will cost you more in the long run.

The responsibility for your health is your own. Hand it off to others with the greatest care.

Appendixes,

Resources,

References,

Index

Appendix A

Symptoms from Inhalation of Mercury Vapor

Acute Exposure

◆ Abdominal disturbances, diarrhea
◆ Behavioral changes (aggressive persona, irritability, shyness, confidence loss, nervousness)
◆ Breathing difficulties, possible pneumonitis with chest pain
◆ Burning sensation in mouth
◆ Deficient performances in everyday actions (cognitive functions)
◆ Dry cough, difficulty swallowing
◆ Fatigue, muscle aches (myalgia)
◆ Flu-like symptoms
◆ Headache
◆ Hypertension (high blood pressure)
◆ Insomnia
◆ Memory or concentration loss ("brain fog")
◆ Nausea
◆ Paresthesias (numbness, tingling) eventually leading to abnormal sensations in hands with abnormal reflexes elsewhere
◆ Tachycardia (rapid heart rate)
◆ Tremors (extremities, eyelids)
◆ Urine production decreased, possible blood in urine
◆ Visual disturbances
◆ Weakness, muscle atrophy (wasting)

Chronic Exposure

◆ Advanced behavioral changes
◆ Alzheimer's disease
◆ Blurred vision
◆ Irritable bowel syndrome (IBS)
◆ Cardiac myopathy (degenerative changes in heart and heart muscles)

- Color vision loss
- Coma
- Poor concentration
- Corneal and lens changes
- Chronic fatigue, fibromyalgia
- Death
- Increase in incidence of infections
- Increase in inflammatory processes
- Decrease infertility, increase in miscarriage incidence
- Poor motor skills
- Muscular Sclerosis
- Increase chance of myocardial infarction (heart attack)
- Nerve responses slowed
- Renal damage
- Shaky speech
- Unsteady walking

Appendix B

The States Respond

As of 2009, many states had passed legislation to protect their citizens from the dangers of mercury.

California

California legislature requires the dentist to provide a dental-materials fact sheet to every new patient and patients of record before performing dental restoration work. The patient must sign an acknowledgement of receipt of the fact sheet.

Under the Health & Safety Code, a lawsuit was filed and won in 2003 against a dentist

> **NOTICE TO PATIENTS**
> **PROPOSITION 65 WARNING:**
> Dental Amalgam, used in many dental fillings, causes exposure to mercury, a chemical known to the state of California to cause birth defects or other reproductive harm.
> Root canal treatments and restorations, including fillings, crowns and bridges, use chemicals known to the state of California to cause cancer.
> The U.S. Food and Drug Administration has studied the situation and approved for use all dental restorative materials.
> Consult your dentist to determine which materials are appropriate for your treatment.

for not revealing that there was mercury in the filings he was placing in patient's teeth. The code applies to mercury dental fillings and states:

> 25249.6. Required Warning Before Exposure To Chemicals Known to Cause Cancer Or Reproductive Toxicity. No person in the course of doing business shall knowingly and intentionally expose any individual to a chemical known to the state to cause cancer or reproductive toxicity without first giving clear and reasonable warning to such individual, except as provided in Section 25249.10.

California legislature recognized the potential of mercury fillings to cause cancer and reproductive toxicity. The consent judgment forced the California Board of Dentistry to assure that patients of dental practices greater than 10 employees were exposed to a poster in the office warning of the danger of mercury fillings.

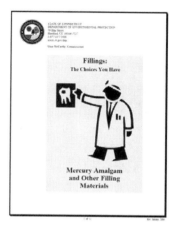

Colorado

Colorado passed legislation to assure a dentist can replace an old mercury amalgam without disciplinary action by the state board of dentistry. This was in response to the "gag order" from state boards of dentistry. Available at:

http://www.state.co.us/gov_dir/leg_dir/olls/sl1997/sl.67.htm

Connecticut

Sections of the Connecticut General Statutes specify:
♦ How mercury amalgam is to be handled, stored and used.
♦ Amalgam separators are mandatory. (see Amalgam Separators)
♦ Each dentist must display the patient fact brochure about the alternatives to mercury fillings, and make a copy available to the patient.

Maine

Maine requires:
♦ Dental amalgam separators must be installed to remove mercury particles before discharging into the local wastewater per a bill effective in the state of Maine. (Legislature of Maine, Chapter 697, Sec.1.38 MRSA §§1661, sub1A and 1B. Available at:
http://www.mainelegislature.org/legis/bills_121st/billtexts/ld069701-1.asp)

New Hampshire

New Hampshire requires that patients be warned about the hazards of mercury in children under the age of 6. A brochure and fact sheet must be available to patients. Dental offices are required to use mercury amalgam separators for removal of mercury before discharge.

New York

New York regulations require amalgam recycling separators for dental offices.

Pennsylvania

Over one and one-half years after the Philadelphia City Council considered and passed the "Mercury in Dentistry" legislation, the Pennsylvania Dental Association (PDA), part of the American Dental Association, is still fighting to prevent patients from knowing what is going to be put in their mouths. The legislation is not to prevent the use of toxic mercury in the mouth (which would be the safest path) but only to *inform the patient* about the materials the dentist is using. The president of the PDA stated "no dentist places mercury in a patient's mouth"—a blatant contradiction of fact that strikes me as immoral and unethical. The Philadelphia Department of Health is becoming aware of the long-term cover-up of mercury and dental amalgam fillings and appears to favor full disclosure to the patient. This would force the dentist to allow informed consent for the patient. Patients would know that mercury was being put in their mouths and could decide if that was what they wanted. Let us hope that City of Philadelphia politicians do what is right for the public.

Resource List

The following list is in no sense intended to be comprehensive. These are simply resources known to me and for that reason, most are in the Pennsylvania area. They may suggest, though, the sort of resources available in your region.

Dentists

Safe dental care: see biosafedentistry
www.biosafedentistry.com
www.donaldrobbinsdmd.com

Safe dentist list:
www.biosafedentistry.com

See the association for safe dentistry:
www.associationforsafedentistry.com

Further Information

www.donaldrobbinsdmd.com
www.toxicteeth.org
www.iaomt.org
www.abcmt.org
www.momsagainstmercury.org
www.protectingyourhealth.com
www.autism.com
www.fluoridealert.org
www.fluorideaction.net

Is your water fluoridated? Go to
http://apps.nccd.cdc.gov/MWF/index.asp

Which fish has more mercury? Go to
http://www.cfsan.fda.gov/~frf/sea-mehg.html

Fluoride content of various foods
http://poisonfluoride.com/pfpc/html/f-_in_food.html

Naturopathic doctors

Kayla Evan, ND
Biogenesis
972 Lincoln Road
Phoenixville, PA 19460-2137
610-933-1982

Bryce Wylde, RNC, DHMHS, HD
Vaughan Medical Centre
9200 Weston Rd.
Vaughan, Ontario, Canada
905-417-2273 x3
www.drwylde.com

Oral Surgeons

Peter Famiglio, DMD
Brandywine Dental Implant and Oral Maxillofacial Surgery
Lionville Professional Center
25 Dowlin Forge Road
Exton, PA 19341
610-363-7000
www.brandywineoralsurgery.com

Pedodontic (Children and Adolescent) Dentistry

Sandra E. Grzybicki, DMD
Paoli West Professional Park
Suite 203
17 Industrial Blvd
Paoli, Pennsylvania 19301-1622
610-647-6688

Physicians (Integrative and Alternative)

Paul Barone, DO
Sharon Barone, DC
Integrated Health and Wellness Center
855 Springdale Drive, Suite 120
Exton, PA 19341
610-524-9520
www.integratedhealthandwellnesscenter.com

Rashid A. Buttar, DO, FAAPM, FACAM, FAAIM
Centers For Advanced Medicine & Clinical Research
9630 Julian Clark Avenue
Huntersville, NC 28078
(704) 895-9355
e-mail: chairman@abcmt.org
www.drbuttar.com

Ira Cantor, MD
Steiner Medical and Therapeutic Center
1220 Valley Forge Road
Phoenixville, PA 19460
610-933-1688

Susan Dallas-Feeney,
DO Integrative Family Medicine
The Commons at Thornbury
42-46 East Street Road
West Chester, PA 19382
610-399-1100

Conrad Maulfair, Jr., DO
Maulfair Medical Center
403 North Main Street
Topton, PA 19562
610-682-2104
www.drmaulfair.com

Alan Vinitsky, MD
Enlightened Medicine
902 Wind River Lane, Suite 201
Gaithersburg, Maryland 20878-1977
301-840-0002

Woodlands Healing Research Center
Harold Buttram, MD, William Kracht, DO, FAAFP,
Robert Schmidt, DO, Nicholas Dimartino, DO
5724 Clymer Road
Quakertown, PA 18951
215-536-1890

Physicians (Holistic)

Peter Prociuk, MD
Classical Homeopathy
Village Hall Clinic
322 North High Street
West Chester, PA 19380
610-701-5702
docRemedy@aol.com

References: Mercury

A Short History of Dentistry

Information about the founding of the first dental school and the first national dental organization, The American Society of Dental Surgeons, in the United States available at:

http://www.fauchard.org/awards/fame8.htm and
http://www.fauchard.org/awards/fame7.htm

Additional details describing dental practices and the position of the founders of The American Society of Dental Surgeons are available in the following articles:

McCauley HB. The first dental college: emergence of dentistry as an autonomous profession. *J Hist Dent*. 2003;51:41-45.

Talbot ES. The chemistry and physiological action of mercury as used in amalgam fillings. *The Ohio State J Dent Sci*. 1882;2(1):1-12.

A Short History of the Tannery Industry

Information about the origin of the phrase "mad as a hatter' is described in *The Mad Hatter*. This information is available at:

http://en.wikipedia.org/w/index.php?title=Mad_Hatter&oldid=121387507

Information about Wernicke's encephalopathy is provided in the following references:

Health A to Z. Korsakoff's syndrome. Available at:
http://www.healthatoz.com/healthatoz/Atoz/common/standard/
transform.jsp?requestURI=/healthatoz/Atoz/ency/
korsakoffs_syndrome.jsp

Alzheimer's Society Information Sheet.

What is Korsakoff's syndrome? Updated October 2008 Available at:
http://www.alzheimers.org.uk/factsheet/438

Korsakoff's syndrome. Available at:
http://en.wikipedia.org/w/
index.php?title=Korsakoff%27s_syndrome&oldid=123713299

SOURCES OF MERCURY EXPOSURE

The following studies measured the amount of mercury in plasma, blood, and urine immediately and several months after simple removal of mercury amalgam dental fillings without precautions.

Bjorkman L, Sandborgh-Englund G, and Ekstrand J. Mercury in saliva and feces after removal of amalgam fillings. *Toxicol Appl Pharmacol.* 1997;FIND VOLUME *Toxicol Appl Pharmacol.* 1997, 144:(1):156-162.

Sandborgh-Englund G, Elinder CG, Langworth S, Schutz A, Ekstrand J. Mercury in biological fluids after amalgam removal. *J Dent Res.* 1998. 77: 615-624.

Molin M, Marklund SL, Bergman B, Nilsson B. Mercury, selenium, and glutathione peroxidase in dental personnel. *Acta Odontol Scand.* 1989. 47:383-390.

Halbach S, Kremers L, Willruth H, Mehl A, Welzl G, Wack FX, Hickel R, Greim H. Systemic transfer of mercury from amalgam fillings before and after cessation of emission. *Environ Res.* 1998;77: 115-123.

Langworth S, Stromberg R. A case of high mercury exposure from dental amalgam. *Eur J Oral Sci.* 1996;104:320-321.

Barregard L, Sallsten G, Jarvholm B. People with high mercury uptake from their own dental amalgam fillings. *Occup Environ Med.* 1995;52:124-128.

Fertilizers

Report from John Gilkeson describing the manufacture, use, and availability of mercury-containing pesticides is available through the United States Environmental Protection Agency:

Gilkeson J. Bureau of Watershed Management, Great Lakes Pollution Prevention and Toxics Reduction. *Mercury Use: Agriculture.* May 1997 report. Available at:

http://www.epa.gov/glnpo/bnsdocs/hgsbook/

Insecticides

Information describing the Teflon controversy and related lawsuits is available through the United States Environmental Protection Agency, Environmental Working Group and DuPont. *EPA's PFOA Investigation.* July 2005 interview.

Fish

Information about the amount of mercury found in various fish and dental mercury fillings assembled by the World Health Organization is available in the following documents:

The World Health Organization, International Programme on Chemical Safety (Environmental Health Criteria 118). *Inorganic mercury.* 1991.

World Health Organization. Concise International Chemical Assessment Document 50, Elemental Mercury and Inorganic Mercury Compounds: Human Health Aspects. 2003. Available at:

http://www.who.int/ipcs/publications/cicad/en/cicad50.pdf

Information about the amount of mercury found in various fish and dental mercury fillings assembled by the Agency for Toxic Substances and Disease Registry is presented in:

United States Department of Health & Human Services, Agency for Toxic Substances and Disease Registry. *Toxicological Profile for Mercury.* March 1999. Available at:

http://www.atsdr.cdc.gov/cercla/97list.html

http://www.atsdr.cdc.gov/toxprofiles/tp46.pdf

Information about the amount of mercury found in various fish assembled by the United States Food and Drug Administration is presented in:

Mercury levels in commercial fish and shellfish. Available at:

http://www.cfsan.fda.gov/~frf/sea-mehg.html

Information about the amount of mercury found in dental mercury fillings is presented in the following articles:

Lorscheider FL, Vimy MJ, Summers AO. Mercury exposure from "silver" tooth fillings: Emerging evidence questions a traditional dental paradigm. *FASEB Journal.* 1995;9:504-508.

Weiner JA, Nylander M. An estimation of the uptake of mercury from amalgam fillings based on urinary excretion of mercury in Swedish subjects. *Sci Total Environ.* 1995;168:255-65.

Björkman L, Sandborgh-Englund G, Ekstrand J. Mercury in salvia and feces after removal of amalgam fillings. *Toxicol Appl Pharmacol.* 1997;144:156-162.

Sandborgh-Englund G, Elinder CG, Johanson G, Lind B, Skare I, Ekstrand J. The absorption, blood levels and excretion of mercury after a single dose of mercury in humans. *Toxicol Appl Pharmacol.* 1998;150(1):146-153.

Data from the following sources were used to generate Graph 1-1

World Health Organization. International Programme on Chemical Safety (Environmental Health Criteria 118). *Inorganic mercury.* 1991.

United States Department of Health & Human Services, Agency for Toxic Substances and Disease Registry. *Toxicological Profile for Mercury.* March 1999. Available at:

http://www.atsdr.cdc.gov/cercla/97list.html

http://www.atsdr.cdc.gov/toxprofiles/tp46.pdf

Zander D, Ewers U, Freier I, Westerweller S, Jermann E, Brockhaus A. [Exposure to mercury in the population. II. Mercury release from amalgam fillings.] *Zentralbl Hyg Umweltmed.* 1990;190:325-334.

Coal Plants

The NESCAUM report, *Mercury Emissions from Coal-Fired Power Plants*, Oct 2003, is available at:

http://www.nescaum.org/documents/rpt031104mercury.pdf/

Thermometers, Thermostats and Other Devices

Study identifying the amount of mercury sold in thermostats in the United States in 2001:

Interstate Mercury Education & Reduction Clearinghouse (IMERC) 2001. *Mercury use in thermostats. Fact sheet. Updated July 2008* Available at:

http://www.newmoa.org/prevention/mercury/imerc/FactSheets/
thermostats.pdf

Report by Environment Canada addressing the amount of mercury in thermometers:

Mercury and the environment. Available at:

http://www.ec.gc.ca/MERCURY/SM/EN/sm-mcp.cfm?SELECT=SM

American Academy of Pediatrics (AAP) recommendation regarding mercury thermometers:

AAP news release. AAP supports elimination of mercury-containing thermometers.

Michael Shannon. Pediatricians, parents urged to stop using mercury thermometers *AAP News*, Jul 2001;19: 21. Available at:

http://aapnews.aappublications.org/cgi/reprint/19/1/
21?maxtoshow=&HITS=10&hits=10&RESULTFORMAT=&fulltext=
thermometers&searchid=1&FIRSTINDEX=0&resourcetype=HWCIT

United States Environmental Protection Agency recommendation regarding mercury thermometers:

Goldman L, Shannon M, et al. Technical report: Mercury in the environment: implications for pediatricians. *Pediatrics*. 2001;108(1):197-205. Available at:
http://aappolicy.aappublications.org/cgi/content/full/pediatrics;108/1/197

Vaccines with Thiomersal

Information about the amount of thimerosal and mercury in vaccines assembled by the Center for Biologicals Evaluation and Research, United States Food and Drug Administration is available in

Thimerosal in vaccines. 2006. Available at:
http://www.fda.gov/cber/vaccine/thimerosal.htm

Report from the National Academy of Sciences to Congress addressing the methylmercury minimal safety dose:

Committee on the Toxicological Effects of Methylmercury, Board of Environmental Studies and Toxicology, National Research Council. *Toxicological Effects of Methylmercury*. Available at:
http://www.nap.edu/catalog/9899.html

Information about adult vaccines containing thimerosal and mercury is available in the following documents:

John Hopkins Bloomberg School of Public Health. *Thimerosal, a mercury-containing preservative used in some vaccines*. July 8, 1999. Available at:
http://www.vaccinesafety.edu/thimerosal.htm.

John Hopkins Bloomberg School of Public Health. *Thimerosal content in some US licensed vaccines*. Oct 16, 2006. Available at:
http://www.vaccinesafety.edu/thi-table.htm.

Troubles Down the Drain

California Assembly Bill 611. *Dental amalgam separators*. Feb 2003. Available at:
http://www.leginfo.ca.gov/pub/03-04/bill/asm/ab_0601-0650/
  ab_611_cfa_20030520_162140_asm_comm.html
http://www.leginfo.ca.gov/pub/03-04/bill/asm/ab_0601-0650/
  ab_611_cfa_20030430_143325_asm_comm.html
http://www.leginfo.ca.gov/pub/03-04/bill/asm/ab_0601-0650/
  ab_611_bill_20030219_introduced.pdf

Information regarding recommendations of the American Dental Association and the Michigan Dental Association are available at:

Environmental Protection Agency Bureau of Watershed Management. Great
  Lakes Pollution Prevention and Toxics Reduction. Draft Wisconsin Mercury Sourcebook: *Dentists, Mercury Use: Dentists*. May 1997. Available at:
http://www.epa.gov/glnpo/bnsdocs/hgsbook/dentist.pdf

Information assembled by the Massachusettes Department of Environmental Protection addressing the use of amalgam separators in dental offices is presented in

Dental amalgam/mercury recycling: About the voluntary program. 2004. Available at:
http://www.mass.gov/dep/service/about08.htm

Information assembled by the City of Palo Alto Regional Water Quality Control Plant addressing the use of amalgam separators in dental offices is presented in

Dental Amalgam Recovery Program, May 2004. Available at:
http://www.cityofpaloalto.org/cleanbay/dental.html

September 7, 2006: Mercury Truth Day

Information addressing the sources of mercury vapor is available in the following documents:

World Health Organization, Department of Protection of the Human Environment. Policy Paper, *Mercury in Health Care*. August 2005. Available at:
http://www.who.int/water_sanitation_health/medicalwaste/
  mercurypolpaper.pdf

Mark Richardson, Environmental Health Directorate, Health Canada. *Assessment of Mercury Exposure and Risks from Dental Amalgam, 1995. Final Report.*

United States Department of Health & Human Services, Agency for Toxic Substances and Disease Registry. *Toxicological Profile for Mercury*. March 1999. Available at:

http://www.atsdr.cdc.gov/cercla/97list.html

http://www.atsdr.cdc.gov/toxprofiles/tp46.pdf

Kingman A, Albertini T, Brown LJ. Mercury concentrations in urine and blood associated with amalgam exposure in the U.S. military population. *Dent Res*. 1998;77:461-471.

Kraub P, Deyhle M. *Field Study on the Mercury Content of Saliva*. 1997. Universitat Tubingen-Institut fur Organische Chemie. 20,000 people tested for mercury level in saliva and health status/symptoms compiled. Available at:

http://www.uni-tuebingen.de/KRAUSS/amalgam.html.

Engqvist A. Speciation of mercury excreted in feces from individuals with amalgam fillings. *Arch Environ Health*. 1998;53:205-213. Available through the Department of Toxicology and Chemistry, Stockholm University, National Institute for Working Life, 1998 at: www.niwl.se/ah/1998-02.html.

Weiner JA, Nylander M. The relationship between mercury concentration in human organs and predictor variables. *Sci Total Environment*. 1993;138:101-115.

Vimy MJ, Lorscheider FL. *J Trace Elem Exper Med*. 1990;3: 111-123.

Barregard L, Sallsten G, Jarvholm B. People with high mercury uptake from their own dental amalgam fillings. *Occup Envir Med*. 1995;52:124-128.

Bjorkman L, Sandborgh-Englund G, Ekstrand J. Mercury in saliva and feces after removal of amalgam fillings. *Toxicol Appl Pharmacol*. 1997;144:156-162.

Berglund A, Molin M. Mercury levels in plasma and urine after removal of all amalgam restorations: the effect of using rubber dams. *Dent Mater*. 1997;13:297-304.

Begerow J, Zander D, Freier I, Dunemann L. Long term mercury excretion in urine after removal of amalgam fillings. *Int Arch Occup Health*. 1994;66:209-212.

Sallsten G, Thoren J, Barregard L, Schutz A, Skarping G. Long term use of chewing gum and mercury exposure from dental amalgam. *J Dental Research*. 1996;75:594-598.

Skare I. Mass balance and systemic uptake of mercury released from dental fillings. *Water, Air, and Soil Pollution*. 1995;80:59-67.

Windham B. Anotated Bibliography: Exposure and Health Effects from Amalgam Fillings. 2000. Over 800 references & 60,000 clinical replacement cases. Available at:
www.flcd.com/fdarevl.html.

Sandborgh-Englund G, Elinder CG, Langworth S, Schutz A, Ekstrand J. Mercury in biological fluids after amalgam removal. *J Dent Res.* 1998;77:615-624.

Aposhian HV. Mobilization of mercury and arsenic in humans by sodium 2,3-dimercapto-1-propane sulfonate (DMPS). *Environ Health Perspect.* 1998;106(Suppl 4):1017-1025.

Aposhian HV. Urinary mercury after administration of 2,3-dimercaptopropane-1-sulfonic acid: correlation with dental amalgam score. *FASEB J.* 1992;6:2472-2476.

Why Did it Take so Long?

Information from the Centers for Devices and Radiological Health, United States Food and Drug Administration addressing release of mercury vapor from mercury-amalgam dental fillings is presented in *Questions and Answers on Dental Amalgam.* Available at:
http://www.fda.gov/cdrh/consumer/amalgams.html

Amalgam Problems I: Off-Gassing and Leaching of Toxic Metals

Information addressing the release of mercury vapor from mercury-amalgam dental fillings is available in the following documents:

Chew CL, Soh G, Lee AS, Yeoh TS. Long-term dissolution of mercury from a non-mercury-releasing amalgam. *Clinical Preventive Dentistry.* 1991;13:5-7.

Vimy MJ, Lorscheided FL. Intra-oral air mercury released from dental amalgam. *J Dent Res.* 1985;64:1069-71.

Tin excesses can be from dental fillings, stannous fluoride in toothpastes or water exposed to brass or tin-containing solders. The organic forms of tin are more toxic and are commonly from herbicide, insecticides or fungicides. Tin can cause headaches (cerebral edema) and suppression of the immune system.

Wilson's disease is caused by excess copper in the body's tissues with

inherent increases in urinary copper excretion. The condition which can be genetic in origin, can also be caused by absorption of copper from water pipes, made worse with the water chlorination process. Symptoms are indicative of liver dysfunction with neurological and blood abnormalities.

Information addressing the release of mercury vapor from mercury-amalgam dental fillings is available from the

World Health Organization, International Programme on Chemical Safety (Environmental Health Criteria 118). *Inorganic mercury.* 1991.

Information addressing the release of mercury vapor from mercury-amalgam dental fillings is available in

Nierenberg DW, Nordgren RE, Chang MB, Siegler RW, Blayney MB, Hochberg F, Toribara TY, Cernichiari E, Clarkson T. Delayed cerebellar disease and death after accidental exposure to dimethylmercury. *N Engl J Med.* 1998;338:1672-1676.

Information addressing the contribution to mercury body burden by mercury-amalgam dental fillings is available in the following documents:

Weiner JA, Nylander M. An estimation of the uptake of mercury from amalgam fillings based on urinary excretion of mercury in Swedish subjects. *Sci Total Environ.* 1995;168:255-265.

United States Department of Health and Human Services, Public Health Service. *Dental amalgam: A scientific review and recommended public health service strategy for research, education and regulation.* Washington, DC. 1993.

Health Canada. *Health Canada position statement on dental amalgam.* 15 September 1997. Update available at:

http://www.hc-sc.gc.ca/dhp-mps/md-im/applic-demande/pubs/ dent_amalgam-eng.php

Information addressing the amount of mercury released from mercury-amalgam dental fillings is presented in the following documents:

Lorscheider FL, Vimy MJ, Summers AO. Mercury exposure from "silver" tooth fillings: Emerging evidence questions a traditional dental paradigm. *FASEB Journal.* 1995;9:504-508.

Vimy MJ, Lorscheider FL. Serial measurements of intra-oral air mercury: estimation of daily dose from dental amalgam. *J Dent Res.* 1985;64:1072-1075.

Information addressing the toxic potential of mercury-amalgam dental fillings is presented in

Wataha JC, Nakajima H, Hanks CT, Okabe T. Correlation of cytotoxicity with element release from mercury and gallium-based dental alloys in vitro. *Dental Materials*. 1994;10:298-303.

Information addressing the absorption of mercury from mercury-amalgam dental fillings is available in the following documents:

Langworth S, Strömberg R. A case of high mercury exposure from dental amalgam. *Eur J Oral Sci.* 1996;104:320-321.

Hanson M, Pleva J. The dental amalgam issue. A review. *Experientia.* 1991;47:9-22.

Jackson GH, Chem BS, Law JD. Quantitative analysis of Hg, Ag, Sn, Cu, Zn and trace elements in amalgam removed from an abutment tooth underneath a gold alloy bridge that had been in vivo for nine plus years. Available at:

http://www.ibiblio.org/amalgam/amalgamtext.html

Measuring Mercury Vapor in the Mouth

Information addressing the effects of mercury from mercury-amalgam dental fillings is presented in

Vimy MJ, Lorscheider FL. Serial measurements of intra-oral air mercury: estimation of daily dose from dental amalgam. *J Dent Res.* 1985;64:1072-1075.

Mercury Vapor Study Results

The data I used to generate graphs 1-2, 1-3, and 1-4 were collected and evaluated statistically. Parameters that could influence data readings include volume of amalgam filling (not just surfaces), variations in mercury content of each filling (usually determined from the original mixed ratio of mercury to alloy), soft tissue interference with a sampling wand (puffy cheeks, large tongue, facial structure), breathing patterns. I am preparing these data for scientific publication.

Information addressing accumulation of mercury from mercury-amalgam dental fillings accumulating in fetuses and children through

their mothers is available in the following documents:

United States Department of Health & Human Services, Agency for Toxic Substances and Disease Registry. *Toxicological Profile for Mercury*. March 1999. Available at:

http://www.atsdr.cdc.gov/cercla/97list.html

http://www.atsdr.cdc.gov/toxprofiles/tp46.pdf

World Health Organization. 2003. Concise International Chemical Assessment Document 50, Elemental Mercury and Inorganic Mercury Compounds: Human Health Aspects. Available at:

http://www.who.int/ipcs/publications/cicad/en/cicad50.pdf

Goldman L, Shannon M, et al. Technical report: Mercury in the environment: implications for pediatricians. *Pediatrics*. 2001;108:197–205. Available at:

http://aappolicy.aappublications.org/cgi/content/full/pediatrics;108/1/197

Maximum Allowable Mercury Levels

The Occupational Safety and Hazard Administration published standards are available through the

Environmental Protection Agency. *Mercury, elemental (CASRN 7439-97-6) IRIS Substance*. Jan 2007. Available at:

http://www.epa.gov/iris/subs/0370.htm, accessed through

http://www.epa.gov/iris/

The National Institute for Occupational Safety and Health (NIOSH) standards are available through

the Center for Disease Control. *Mercury compounds [except (organo) alkyls]. NIOSH pocket guide to chemical hazards*. No.2005-149. Sep 2005. Available at:

http://www.cdc.gov/niosh/npg/npgd0383.html

TWA or time-weighted average is the "allowable" exposure concentration over a normal 8-hour workday or a 40-hour work week. Above this level the studies reviewed by the organization showed adverse health effects appearing.

The American Conference of Governmental Industrial Hygienists standards are available through the

United States Department of Labor. *Occupational Safety and Health Guideline for Mercury Vapor*. Sep 1996. Available at:

http://www.osha.gov/SLTC/healthguidelines/mercuryvapor/
   recognition.html

TLV or threshold limit value is the concentration to which workers can be exposed without adverse health effects.

The Environmental Protection Agency standards are available through the

Environmental Protection Agency. *Mercury, elemental (CASRN 7439-97-6) IRIS Substance.* Jan 2007. Available at:
http://www.epa.gov/iris/subs/0370.htm, accessed through
http://www.epa.gov/iris/

Agency for Toxic Substances and Disease Registry standards are available through the

United States Department of Health & Human Services, Agency for Toxic Substances and Disease Registry. *Minimal risk levels (MRLs) for hazardous substances.* Dec 2006. Available at:
http://www.atsdr.cdc.gov/mrls/index.html

The standards set by Health Canada are available through

Mark Richardson, Environmental Health Directorate, Health Canada. *Assessment of Mercury Exposure and Risks from Dental Amalgam, 1995. Final Report.*

Mercury Exposure: The Bottom Line

Information addressing non-residential limits for mercury levels is available in the following documents:

United States Department of Health and Human Services. State of Kentucky Health Consultation. *Mercury Contamination in Indoor Air.* Mar 2005. Available at:
http://www.atsdr.cdc.gov/HAC/pha/StateofKYMercury031505-KY/
   StateofKYMercury031505-KY.pdf

Department of Community Health. Suggested Action Levels for Indoor Mercury Vapor in Michigan. Nov 2003. Available at:
http://www.michigan.gov/documents/
   mdch_MercuryCleanupGuidance_85690_7.pdf

New Jersey's side of the toxic day-care story.
Philly.com home page. 9 Aug 2006.

Hefler J. Mercury effects linger, lawyer says. *Philadelphia Inquirer* 15 Sep 2006. Page B01.

Measuring Mercury Levels in the Body

Information addressing the urine challenge test is available in

Gonzalez-Ramirez D, Maiorino RM, Zuniga-Charles M, Xu Z, Hurlbut KM, Junco-Munoz P, Aposhian MM, Dart RC, Diaz Gama JH, Echeverria, D. Sodium 2,3-dimercaptopropane-1-sulfonate challenge test for mercury in humans: II. Urinary mercury, porphyrins and neurobehavioral changes of dental workers in Monterrey, Mexico. *J Pharmacol Exp Ther.* 1995;272:264-274.

The Baddest Tattoo

Information addressing the mercury concentration of tissues is presented in the

United States Department of Health & Human Services, Agency for Toxic Substances and Disease Registry. *Toxicological Profile for Mercury.* March 1999. Available at:
http://www.atsdr.cdc.gov/cercla/97list.html
http://www.atsdr.cdc.gov/toxprofiles/tp46.pdf

Information addressing lichen planus is presented in

Smart ER, Macleod RI, Lawrence CM. Resolution of lichen planus following removal of amalgam restorations in patients with proven allergy to mercury salts: a pilot study. *Br Dent J.* 1995;178: 108-112.

The Toxic Dental Office

Information addressing exposure of individuals to mercury through mercury-amalgam dental fillings is available in the following documents:

World Health Organization, Department of Protection of the Human Environment. August 2005. Policy Paper, Mercury in Health Care. Available at:
http://www.who.int/water_sanitation_health/medicalwaste/
mercurypolpaper.pdf

Mark Richardson, Environmental Health Directorate, Health Canada. Assessment of Mercury Exposure and Risks from Dental Amalgam, 1995. Final Report.

United States Department of Health & Human Services, Agency for Toxic Substances and Disease Registry. *Toxicological Profile for Mercury*. March 1999. Available at:

http://www.atsdr.cdc.gov/cercla/97list.html

http://www.atsdr.cdc.gov/toxprofiles/tp46.pdf

Kingman A, Albertini T, Brown L J. Mercury concentrations in urine and blood associated with amalgam exposure in the U.S. military population. *Dent Res.* 1998;77:461-471.

Kraub P, Deyhle M, Maier KH, Roller HD. Field study on the mercury content of saliva. *Heavy Metal Bull.* 1996;3.

Kraub P, Deyhle M. Field Study on the Mercury Content of Saliva. 1997. Universitat Tubingen-Institut fur Organische Chemie. 20,000 people tested for mercury level in saliva and health status/symptoms compiled. Available: http://www.uni-tuebingen.de/KRAUSS/amalgam.html.

Engqvist A. Speciation of mercury excreted in feces from individuals with amalgam fillings. *Arch Environ Health.* 1998;53:205-213. Department of Toxicology and Chemistry, Stockholm University, National Institute for Working Life, 1998. Available at:

www.niwl.se/ah/1998-02.html

Weiner JA, Nylander M. The relationship between mercury concentration in human organs and predictor variables. *Sci Total Environment.* 1993;138:101-115.

Vimy MJ, Lorscheider FL. *J Trace Elem Exper Med.* 1990;3: 111-123.

Barregard L, Sallsten G, Jarvholm B. People with high mercury uptake from their own dental amalgam fillings. *Occup Environ Med.* 1995;52(2):124-128.

Bjorkman L, Sandborgh-Englund G, and Ekstrand J. Mercury in saliva and feces after removal of amalgam fillings. *Toxicol Appl Pharmacol.* 1997;144:156-162.

Berglund A, Molin M. Mercury levels in plasma and urine after removal of all amalgam restorations: the effect of using rubber dams. *Dent Mater.* 1997;13:297-304.

Begerow J, Zander D, Freier I, Dunemann L. Long term mercury excretion in urine after removal of amalgam fillings. *Int Arch Occup Health.* 1994;66:209-212.

Sallsten G, Thoren J, Barregard L, Schutz A, Skarping G. Long term use of chewing gum and mercury exposure from dental amalgam. *J Dental Research*. 1996;75:594-598.

Skare I. Mass balance and systemic uptake of mercury released from dental fillings. *Water, Air, and Soil Pollution*. 1995;80:59-67.

Windham B. Mercury exposure levels from amalgam dental fillings; Documentation of Mechanisms by Which Mercury Causes over 40 Chronic Health Conditions; Results of Replacement of Amalgam Fillings; and Occupational Effects on Dental Staff. Rockville, MD: US FDA; 2002. Available at:

http://www.fda.gov/OHRMS/DOCKETS/dailys/02/Sep02/091602/80027dde.pdf

Sandborgh-Englund G, Elinder CG, Langworth S, Schutz A, Ekstrand J. Mercury in biological fluids after amalgam removal. *J Dent Res*. 1998;77(4):615-624.

Aposhian HV. Mobilization of mercury and arsenic in humans by sodium 2,3-dimercapto-1-propane sulfonate (DMPS). *Environ Health Perspect*. 1998;106(Suppl 4):1017-1025.

Aposhian HV. Urinary mercury after administration of 2,3-dimercaptopropane-1-sulfonic acid: correlation with dental amalgam score. *FASEB J*. 1992;6:2472-2476.

Zander D, Ewers U, Freier I, Westerweller S, Jermann E, Brockhaus A. [Exposure to mercury in the population. II. Mercury release from amalgam fillings.] *Zentralbl Hyg Umweltmed*. 1990;190:325-334.

Molin M, Marklund SL, Bergman B, Nilsson B. Mercury, selenium, and glutathione peroxidase in dental personnel. *Acta Odontol Scand*. 1989. 47:383-390.

The Toxic Dentist Is Everywhere

Information addressing mercury levels in the urine of dentists is presented in the following documents:

Naleway C, Chou HN, Muller T, et al. On-site screening for urinary Hg concentrations and correlation with glomerular and renal tubular function. *J Public Health Dent*, 1991;51(1):12-17.

Naleway C, Muller T, Sakaguchi R, et al. Urinary mercury levels in U.S. dentists, 1975-1983: Review of health assessment program. *J Am Dent Assoc*. 1985;111:37-42.

Information addressing symptoms related to mercury exposure and metabolism is presented in the following documents:

Sandborgh-Englund G, Elinder CG, Langworth S, et al. Mercury in biological fluids after amalgam removal. *J Dent Res.* 1998;77(4):615-24

Ekstrand J, Bjorkman L, etal. Toxicological aspects on the release and systemic uptake of mercury from dental amalgam. *Eur J Oral Sci.* 1998;106(2 pr 2):678-86.

Information addressing mercury exposure of dentists is available in the following documents:

Ayyadurai K, Krishnashamy V. A study of mercury concentration in nails, hair, and urine of dentists, dental assistants and non-dental personnel. *J Environ Biol.* 1988;9(3):281-282.

Skare I, Bergstroem T, Engqvist A, et al. Mercury exposure of different origins among dentists and dental nurses. *Scand J Work Environ Health.* 1990;16:340-347.

Nylander M, Friberg L, Eggleston D, et al. Mercury accumulation in tissues from dental staff and controls in relation to exposure. *Swed Dent J.* 1989;13(6):235-243.

Nylander M, Weiner J. Mercury and selenium concentrations and their interrelations in organs from dental staff and the general-population. *Br J Ind Med.* 1991;48(11):729-734.

Vimy MJ, Lorscheided FL. Intra-oral air mercury released from dental amalgam. *J Dent Res.* 1985;64(8):1069-71.

Vimy MJ, Lorscheider FL. Serial measurements of intra-oral air mercury :estimation of daily dose from dental amalgam. *J Dent Res.* 1985;64(80:1072-5.

Molin M, Marklund SL, Bergman B, Nilsson B. Mercury, selenium, and glutathione peroxidase in dental personnel. *Acta Odontol Scand.* 1989. 47:383-390.

Information addressing the results of urine challenge tests in dentists is presented in the following documents:

Naleway C, Chou HN, Muller T, et al. On-site screening for urinary Hg concentrations and correlation with glomerular and renal tubular function. *J Public Health Dent.* 1991;51(1):12-17.

Gilkeson J. Bureau of Watershed Management, Great Lakes Pollution Prevention and Toxics Reduction. Environmental Protection Agency. *Mercury Use: Agriculture.* May 1997. Available:

http://www.epa.gov/glnpo/bnsdocs/hgsbook/agr.pdf

Gonzalez-Ramirez D, Maiorino RM, Zuniga-Charles M, Xu Z, Hurlbut KM, Junco-Munoz P, Aposhian MM; Dart RC, Diaz Gama JH, Echeverria D et al. Sodium 2,3-dimercaptopropane-1-sulfonate challange test for mercury in humans: II. Urinary mercury, porphyrins and neurobehavioral changes of dental workers in Monterrey, Mexico. *J Pharmacol Exp Ther.* 1995;272(1):264-274.

Information addressing the neurological effects and risk of exposure to mercury in dentists is presented in the following documents:

Ngim CH, Foo SC, Boey KW, et al. Chronic neurobehavioural effects of elemental mercury in dentists. *Br J Ind Med.* 1992;49(11):782-790.

Shapiro IM, Sumner AJ, Spitz LK, et al. Neurophysiological and neuropsychological function in mercury exposed dentists. *Lancet.* 1982;1:1147-1150.

Echeverria D, Heyer NJ, Martin MD, et al. Behavioral effects of low-level exposure to elemental Hg among dentists. *Neurotoxicol Teratol.* 1995 17(2):161-8.

Escheverria D, Hever N, Martin MD, Naleway CA, Woods JS Bittner AC; Behavioral effects of low level exposure to mercury among dentists. *Neurotxicol Teratol.* 1995;17:161-168.

Shapiro IM, Cornblath DR, Sumner AJ, et al. Neurophysiological and neuropsychological function in mercury-exposed dentists. *Lancet.* 1982;1:1147-1150.

The Toxic Dental Assistant Is Everywhere

California Assembly Bill 611, Dental amalgam separators, Feb 2003
http://www.leginfo.ca.gov/pub/03-04/bill/asm/ab_0601-0650/
ab_611_cfa_20030520_162140_asm_comm.html
http://www.leginfo.ca.gov/pub/03-04/bill/asm/ab_0601-0650/
ab_611_cfa_20030430_143325_asm_comm.html
http://www.leginfo.ca.gov/pub/03-04/bill/asm/ab_0601-0650/
ab_611_bill_20030219_introduced.pdf

Information addressing accumulation of mercury from mercury-amalgam dental fillings accumulating in fetuses and children through their mothers is presented in

Goldman L, Shannon M, et al. Technical report: Mercury in the environment: implications for pediatricians. *Pediatrics.* 2001;108(1):197-205.
http://aappolicy.aappublications.org/cgi/content/full/pediatrics;108/1/197

Information addressing the risks associated with exposure to mercury from mercury-amalgam dental fillings for dental assistants and dentists is available in the following documents:

Rowland AS, Baird DD, Weinberg CR, et al. The effect of occupational exposure to mercury vapour on the fertility of female dental assistants [see comments]. *Occup Environ Med.* 1994; 51(1):28-34.

Sikorski R, Juszkiewicz T, Paszkowski T, et al. Women in dental surgeries: Reproductive hazards in occupational exposure to metallic mercury. *Int Arch Occup Environ Health.* 1987; 59:551-557.

Gerhard I, Monga B, Waldbrenner A, Runnebaum B Heavy metals and fertility. *J Toxicol Environ Health.* 1998;21;54(8):593-611.

Liang LI, Brooks RJ. Mercury reactions in the human mouth with dental amalgams. *Water, Air, and Soil Pollution.* 1995 80:103-07.

Sellars WA, Sellars Jr R, Liang L, Hefley JD. Methyl mercury in dental amalgams in the human mouth. *J Nutri Envir Med.* 1996 6:33-36.

The Toxic Dental Office Is Everywhere

Information addressing the risk of exposure to mercury in dental offices which do not place mercury-amalgam dental fillings is presented in

Ekstrand, J., et al., Toxicological aspects on the release and systemic uptake of mercury from dental amalgam. *Eur J Oral Sci.* 1998;106(2 Pt 2): 678-86.

The Toxic Dental Patient Is Everywhere

Information addressing the half-life of mercury is presented in

Sandborgh-Englund G, Elinder CG, Langworth S, Schutz A, Ekstrand J. Mercury in biological fluids after amalgam removal. *J Dent Res.* 1998;77(4):615-624.

Out with the Old

Information addressing the reduction of mercury in body fluids following removal of mercury-amalgam dental fillings is presented in following documents:

Sandborgh-Englund G, Elinder CG, Langworth S, Schutz A, Ekstrand J. Mercury in biological fluids after amalgam removal. *J Dent Res.* 1998;77(4):615-624.

Molin M, Marklund SL, Bergman B, Nilsson B. Mercury, selenium, and glutathione peroxidase in dental personnel. *Acta Odontol Scand.* 1989. 47:383-390.

Halbach S, Kremers L, Willruth H, Mehl A, Welzl G, Wack F X, Hickel R, Greim H. Systemic transfer of mercury from amalgam fillings before and after cessation of emission. *Environ Res.* 1998;77(2):115-123.

Langworth S, Stromberg R. A case of high mercury exposure from dental amalgam. *Eur J Oral Sci.* 1996;104(3):320-321.

Barregard L, Sallsten G, Jarvholm B. People with high mercury uptake from their own dental amalgam fillings. *Occup Environ Med.* 1995;52(2):124-128.

Information addressing improvements in patient health status and well being following removal of mercury-amalgam dental fillings is available in the following documents:

Prochazkova J, Sterzl I, Kucerova H, Bartova J, Stejskal VD. The beneficial effect of amalgam replacement on health in patients with autoimmunity. *Neuro Endocrinol Lett.* 2004;25(3):211-8.

Lindh U, Hudecek R, Danersund A, Eriksson S, Lindvall A. Removal of dental amalgam and other metal alloys supported by antioxidant therapy alleviates symptoms and improves quality of life in patients with amalgam-associated ill health. *Neuro Endocrinol Lett.* 2002. 23(5-6):459-482.

Information addressing impact of mercury-amalgam dental filling material to tooth structure or dental crowns is presented in

Jackson GH, Chem BS, Law JD. Quantitative analysis of Hg, Ag, Sn, Cu, Zn and trace elements in amalgam removed from an abutment tooth underneath a gold alloy bridge that had been in vivo for nine plus years. *Available at:*

http://www.ibiblio.org/amalgam/amalgamtext.html

But Safely

Information about the International Academy of Oral Medicine and Toxicology is available at:
http://www.iaomt.org

Information addressing the use of latex dams during removal of dental fillings is presented in

Kremers L, Halbach S Willruth H, Mehl A, Welzl G, Wack FX, Hickel R, Greim H. Effect of rubber dam on mercury exposure during amalgam removal. *Eur J Oral Sci*. 1999. 107(3):202-207.

Mercury Affects the Whole Body

Information addressing the standards for mercury exposure set by the World Health Organization are available through the

World Health Organization. International Programme on Chemical Safety (Environmental Health Criteria 118). *Inorganic mercury*. 1991.

Information addressing the conversion of mercury to methylmercury is presented in

Lindh U, Carlmark B, Gronquist SO, Lindvall A. Metal exposure from amalgam alters the distribution of trace elements in blood cells and plasma. *Clin Chem Lab Med*. 2001;39(2):134-142.

Information addressing the risk to pregnant women, nursing mothers, fetuses, and newborns is presented in the following documents:

NESCAUM. Mercury Emissions from Coal-Fired Power Plants. Oct 2003. Available at:

http://www.nescaum.org/documents/rpt031104mercury.pdf/

Oskarsson A, Palminger Hallen I, Sundberg J. Exposure to toxic elements via breast milk. *Analyst*. 1995;120(3):765-770.

Soederstroem S, Fredriksson A, Dencker L & Ebendal T. The effect of mercury vapour on cholinergic neurons in the fetal brain: studies on the expression of nerve growth factor and its low- and high-affinity receptors. *Dev Brain Res*. 1995;85(1):96-108.

Goldman L, Shannon M, et al. Technical report: Mercury in the environment: implications for pediatricians. *Pediatrics*. 2001;108(1):197-205. Available at: http://aappolicy.aappublications.org/cgi/content/full/pediatrics;108/1/197

Mercury Poisoning: Why Some and Not Others?

Information addressing an individual's ability to excrete toxins is presented in the following documents:

Langworth S, Stromberg R. A case of high mercury exposure from dental amalgam. *Eur J Oral Sci.* 1996;104(3):320-321.

Needleman, HL. Mercury in dental amalgam—a neurotoxic risk? *JAMA.* 2006;295(15):1835-1836.

Echeverria D, Woods JS, Heyer NJ, Rohlman D, Farin FM, Li T, Garabedian CE. The association between a genetic polymorphism of coproporphyrinogen oxidase, dental mercury exposure and neurobehavioral response in humans. *Neurotoxicol Teratol.* 2006;28(1):39-48.

How Mercury Affects the Body's Various Systems

The Cardiovascular System

Information addressing the impact of mercury on the cardiovascular system is presented in the following documents:

United States Department of Health & Human Services, Agency for Toxic Substances and Disease Registry. *Toxicological Profile for Mercury.* March 1999. Available at:

http://www.atsdr.cdc.gov/cercla/97list.html

http://www.atsdr.cdc.gov/toxprofiles/tp46.pdf

Nierenberg DW, Nordgren RE, Chang MB, Siegler RW, Blayney MB, Hochberg F, Toribara TY, Cernichiari E, Clarkson T. Delayed cerebellar disease and death after accidental exposure to dimethylmercury. *N Engl J Med.* 1998;338:1672-1676.

Salonen JT, Seppanen K, Nyyssonen K, Korpela H, Kauhanen J, Kantola M, Tuomilehto J, Esterbauer H, Tatzber F, Salonen R. Intake of mercury from fish, lipid peroxidation, and the risk of myocardial infarction and coronary, cardiovascular, and any death in eastern Finnish men. *Circulation.* 1995;91:645-655.

Frustaci, A., Magnavita N, Chimenti C, Caldarulo M, Sabbioni E, Pietra R, Cellini C, Possati GF, Maseri A. Marked elevation of myocardial trace elements in idiopathic dilated cardiomyopathy compared with secondary cardiac dysfunction. *J Am Coll Cardiol.* 1999;33:1578-1583.

de Assis GP, Silva CE, Stefanon I, Vassallo DV. Effects of small concentrations of mercury on the contractile activity of the rat ventricular myocardium. *Comp Biochem Physiol C Toxicol Pharmacol.* 2003;134:375-383.

The Gastrointestinal System

Information addressing the impact of mercury on the gastrointestinal system is presented in the following documents:

United States Department of Health & Human Services, Agency for Toxic Substances and Disease Registry. *Toxicological Profile for Mercury*. March 1999. Available at:

http://www.atsdr.cdc.gov/cercla/97list.html

http://www.atsdr.cdc.gov/toxprofiles/tp46.pdf

Nierenberg DW, Nordgren RE, Chang MB, Siegler RW, Blayney MB, Hochberg F, Toribara TY, Cernichiari E, Clarkson T. Delayed cerebellar disease and death after accidental exposure to dimethylmercury. *N Engl J Med*. 1998;338:1672-1676.

The Immune System

Information addressing the impact of mercury on the immune system is presented in the following documents:

Moszczynski P, Lisiewica J, Bartus R, et al. Lymphocytes T and NK cells in men occupationally exposed to mercury vapors. *Int J Occup Med Environ Health*. 1995;8:49-56.

Hirsch F, Kuhn J, Ventura M, Vial MC, Fournie G, Druet P. Production of monoclonal antibodies. *J Immunol*. 1986;136:3272-3276.

Hultman P, Johansson U, Turley Sj, Lindh U, Enestrom S, Pollard KM. Adverse immunological effects and autoimmunity induced by dental amalgam and alloy in mice. *FASEB J*. 1994;8:1183-1190.

Biagazzi M, Pierlguigi E. Autoimmunity and heavy metals. *Lupus*. 1994;3:449-453.

Warfvinge K, Hansson H, Hultman P. Systemic autoimmunity due to mercury vapor exposure in genetically susceptible mice: dose-response studies. *Toxicol Appl Pharmacol*. 1995;132:299-309.

Escheverria D, Hever N, Martin MD, Naleway CA, Woods JS Bittner AC. Behavioral effects of low level exposure to mercury among dentists. *Neurotxicol Teratol*. 1995;17:161-168.

Prochazkova J, Sterzl I, Kucerova H, Bartova J, Stejskal VD. The beneficial effect of amalgam replacement on health in patients with autoimmunity. *Neuro Endocrinol Lett*. 2004;25:211-218.

Halbach S, Kremers L, Willruth H, Mehl A, Welzl G, Wack FX, Hickel R, Greim H. Systemic transfer of mercury from amalgam fillings before and after cessation of emission. *Environ Res.* 1998;77(2):115-123.

Langworth S, Strömberg R. A case of high mercury exposure from dental amalgam. *Eur J Oral Sci.* 1996;104:320-321.

Barregård L, Sällsten G, Järvholm B. People with high mercury uptake from their own dental amalgam fillings. *Occup Environ Med.* 1995;52:124-128.

The Neurological System

Information addressing the impact of mercury on the neurological system is presented in the following documents:

World Health Organization. 2003. *Concise International Chemical Assessment Document 50, Elemental Mercury and Inorganic Mercury Compounds: Human Health Aspects.* Available at:

http://www.who.int/ipcs/publications/cicad/en/cicad50.pdf

Nierenberg DW, Nordgren RE, Chang MB, Siegler RW, Blayney MB, Hochberg F, Toribara TY, Cernichiari E, Clarkson T. Delayed cerebellar disease and death after accidental exposure to dimethylmercury. *N Engl J Med.* 1998;338:1672-1676.

Pendergrass JC, Haley BE. Inhibition of brain tubulin-guanosine 5'-triphosphate interactions by mercury: similarity to observations in Alzheimer's diseased brain. *Met Ions Biol Syst.* 1997;34:461-478.

Pendergrass, JC, Haley BE, Vimy MJ, Winfield SA, Lorscheider FL. Mercury vapor inhalation inhibits binding of GTP to tubulin in rat brain: similarity to a molecular lesion in Alzheimer diseased brain. *Neurotoxicology.* 1997;18:315-324.

Thompson CM, Markesbery WR, Ehmann WD, Mao YX, Vance DE. Regional brain trace-element studies in Alzheimer's disease. *Neurotoxicology.* 1988;9:1-7.

Ngim, CH, Devathasan, G. Epidemiologic study on the association between body burden mercury level and idiopathic Parkinson's disease. *Neuroepidemiology.* 1989;8:128-141.

Chang YC, Yeh CY, Wang JD. Subclinical neurotoxicity of mercury vapor revealed by a multimodality evoked potential study of chloralkali workers. *Am J Ind Med.* 1995;27:271-279.

United States Department of Labor. *Occupational Safety and Health Guideline for Mercury Vapor*. 1996. Available at:
http://www.osha.gov/SLTC/healthguidelines/mercuryvapor/recognition.html

Hathaway GJ, PN, Hughes JP, and Fischman ML. *Proctor and Hughes' chemical hazards of the workplace*. 1991. 3rd ed. New York, NY: Van Nostrand Reinhold.

Bagedahl-Strindlund M, Ilie M, Furhoff AK, Tomson Y, Larsson KS, Sandborgh-Englund G, Torstenson B, Wretlind K. A multidisciplinary clinical study of patients suffering from illness associated with mercury release from dental restorations: psychiatric aspects. *Acta Psychiatrica Scandinavica*. 1997;96(6):475–482.

Siblerud TL, Kienholz E. Evidence that mercury from silver dental fillings may be an etiological factor in reduced nerve conduction velocity in multiple sclerosis patients. *J Orthomol Med*. 1997;12:169-172.

Siblerud RL, Kienholz E. Evidence that mercury from silver dental fillings may be an etiological factor in multiple sclerosis. *Sci Total Environ*. 1994;15:142:191-205.

The Ophthalmic System

United States Department of Labor. *Occupational Safety and Health Guideline for Mercury Vapor*. 1996. Available at:
http://www.osha.gov/SLTC/healthguidelines/mercuryvapor/recognition.html

Cavalleri, A, et al. Colour vision loss in workers exposed to elemental mercury vapour. *Toxicol Lett*. 1995;77(1-3):351-356.

Altmann L, et al. Visual functions in 6-year-old children in relation to lead and mercury levels. *Neurotoxicol Teratol*. 1998;20:9-17.

Grant, WM. *Toxicology of the eye*. 3rd ed. Springfield, IL: Charles C Thomas. 1986.

The Renal System

Information addressing the impact of mercury on the renal system is presented in the following documents:

United States Department of Health & Human Services, Agency for Toxic Substances and Disease Registry. *Toxicological Profile for Mercury*. March 1999. Available at:

http://www.atsdr.cdc.gov/cercla/97list.html

http://www.atsdr.cdc.gov/toxprofiles/tp46.pdf

Nierenberg DW, Nordgren RE, Chang MB, Siegler RW, Blayney MB, Hochberg F, Toribara TY, Cernichiari E, Clarkson T. Delayed cerebellar disease and death after accidental exposure to dimethylmercury. *N Engl J Med.* 1998;338:1672-1676.

Nylander, M, Friberg L, and Lind B. Mercury concentrations in the human brain and kidneys in relation to exposure from dental amalgam fillings. *Swed Dent J.* 1987.11:179-187.

Boyd, ND, et al. Mercury from dental "silver" tooth fillings impairs sheep kidney function. *Am J Physiol.* 1991;261(4 Pt 2):R1010-1014.

The Reproductive System

Information addressing the impact of mercury on the reproductive system is presented in the following document:

World Health Organization. 2003. *Concise International Chemical Assessment Document 50, Elemental Mercury and Inorganic Mercury Compounds: Human Health Aspects.* Available at:

http://www.who.int/ipcs/publications/cicad/en/cicad50.pdf

The Respiratory System

Information addressing the impact of mercury on the respiratory system is presented in the following documents:

Nierenberg DW, Nordgren RE, Chang MB, Siegler RW, Blayney MB, Hochberg F, Toribara TY, Cernichiari E, Clarkson T. Delayed cerebellar disease and death after accidental exposure to dimethylmercury. *N Engl J Med.* 1998;338:1672-1676.

United States Department of Labor, *Occupational Safety and Health Guideline for Mercury Vapor,* 1996. Available at:

http://www.osha.gov/SLTC/healthguidelines/mercuryvapor/recognition.html

Hathaway GJ, PN, Hughes JP, and Fischman ML. *Proctor and Hughes' chemical hazards of the workplace.* 3rd ed. New York, NY: Van Nostrand Reinhold. 1991.

Protecting Yourself in the Dentist's Office

Information addressing the risks to pregnant women and fetuses associated with removal of mercury-amalgam dental fillings is presented in the following documents:

United States Department of Health & Human Services, Agency for Toxic Substances and Disease Registry. *Toxicological Profile for Mercury*. March 1999. Available at:

http://www.atsdr.cdc.gov/cercla/97list.html

http://www.atsdr.cdc.gov/toxprofiles/tp46.pdf

Goldman L, SM, et al. Technical report: Mercury in the environment: implications for pediatricians. *Pediatrics*. 108:197-205. Available at:

http://www.cispimmunize.org/pro/pdf/

MercuryinEnvironmentImpforPeds.pdf

References: Other Dental Metals:

Information about gold, platinum, and organo-platinum compounds can be found at the following websites:

http://www.fda.gov/OHRMS/DOCKETS/dailys/03/Nov03/111903/03p-
0530-cp00001-Exhibit-Tab-O-vol1.pdf

http://jpet.aspetjournals.org/cgi/content/abstract/211/3/531

http://www.neuro.wustl.edu/NEUROMUSCULAR/nother/
toxic.htm#cis-platinum

Information from the Identalloy® Council about the metals in alloys used in dental fillings is available at the following websites:

http://www.identalloy.org/PDFs/Brochure_Identalloy_Gold.pdf

http://www.identalloy.org/

Information about the potential side effects beryllium may cause is available at the following websites:

http://www.osha.gov/SLTC/beryllium/recognition.html

http://www.atsdr.cdc.gov/toxprofiles/phs4.html

http://ntp.niehs.nih.gov/ntp/roc/eleventh/profiles/s022bery.pdf

Information about the potential side effects boron may cause is available at the following websites:

http://www.atsdr.cdc.gov/tfacts26.html

http://www.epa.gov/iris/subst/0410.htm

Information about the potential side effects aluminum may cause is available at the following site:

http://www.osha.gov/SLTC/healthguidelines/aluminum/
recognition.html#healthhazard

Information about the potential side effects nickel may cause is available at the following websites:

http://www.cdc.gov/niosh/npg/npgd0445.html

http://www.atsdr.cdc.gov/tfacts15.html#bookmark01

Information about the potential side effects iron may cause is available at the following website:

http://www.cdc.gov/ncbddd/hemochromatosis/

Information about the potential side effects molybdenum may cause is available at the following website:

http://www.cdc.gov/niosh/pel88/7439-98.html

Information about the potential side effects lithium may cause is available at the following websites:

http://www.oehha.ca.gov/public_info/pdf/
    Lithium%20Fact%20Sheet%20Meth%20Labs%2010'03'.pdf
http://www.lenntech.com/Periodic-chart-elements/Li-en.htm

Information about the potential side effects palladium may cause is available at the following websites and sources:

http://www.lenntech.com/Periodic-chart-elements/Pd-en.htm

Blaurock-Busch E. Palladium.
http://www.mercuryexposure.org/index.php?article_id=230

W Moore, D Hysell, L Hall, K Campbell, and J Stara. Preliminary studies on the toxicity and metabolism of palladium and platinum. *Environ Health Perspect.* 1975;10:63–71.

Information about the potential side effects copper is available at the following websites:

Public Wilson L. Copper Toxicity Syndrome
http://drlwilson.com/Articles/copper_toxicity_syndrome.htm and
http://www.drlwilson.com/read%20articles.htm

Health Statement for Copper, ATSDR Sept 2004.
http://www.atsdr.cdc.gov/toxprofiles/phs132.html#bookmark05

The Facts on Copper. Dartmouth Toxic Metals Research Program 2001.
http://www.dartmouth.edu/~toxmetal/TXQAcu.shtml

References: Fluoride

Fluorogate

Information about the studies conducted to test the safety of fluoride are available through the

Centers for Disease Control in *Achievements in Public Health, 1900-1999: Fluoridation of Drinking Water to Prevent Dental Caries.* MMWR Weekly. October 22, 1999;48(41);933-940. Available at:
http://www.cdc.gov/mmwR/preview/mmwrhtml/mm4841a1.htm

Information about Program F is available at
http://www.fluoridealert.org/deepwater.htm

The abstract of the study addressing the view society has of the appearance of an individual's teeth, authored by Brian A. Burt, MPH, PhD of the University of Michigan, was presented at the Dietary Fluoride Supplement Conference of the American Dental Association; the meeting was held in Chicago, Ill in January 1994.

Some of Dr. Dean's work is presented by Peter Meiers in

The History of Fluorine, Fluoride and Fluoridation. Questionable Fluoride Safety Studies: Bartlett vs. Cameron & Newburgh vs. Kingston. Available:
http://www.fluoride-history.de/bartlett.htm

More information about the hearing before the House of Representatives on the topic of fluoridation of water supplies of available at the following references:

Peter Meiers. *The History of Fluorine, Fluoride and Fluoridation. Questionable Fluoride Safety Studies: Bartlett vs. Cameron & Newburgh vs. Kingston.* Available at:
http://www.fluoride-history.de/bartlett.htm

A. L. Miller in *Testimony of David B. Ast representing the American Public Health Association.* Hearings before the House Select Committee to investigate the use of chemicals in foods and cosmetics. House of Representatives, 82nd Congress, 2nd session, pursuant to House Resolution 74 and House Resolution 447, page 159. Washington 1952.

Fluoridation: the "Official" Levels

More information about the early identification of dental fluorosis as a marker of the toxicity of fluoride is available at
http://www.fluoridealert.org/health/epa/memos/white-thurmonod1979.pdf

What's in a Label?

Information about the amount of fluoride in bottled water is available from the Centers for Disease Control in

Recommendations for Using Fluoride to Prevent and Control Dental Caries in the United States. MMWR. Aug 17, 2001;50(RR14):1–42. Available at: http://www.cdc.gov/mmwr/preview/mmwrhtml/rr5014a1.htm

The Battle Continues

Information about Canadian citizens' concerns and actions regarding fluoridation of their water supplies is presented in

Calgary, Canada lawsuits and debate over water fluoridation. Available at: http://www.fluoridation.com/
news.htm#Health%20adviser%20warns%20of%20possible%20
fluoride%20lawsuits

Information about the studies evaluating the safety of fluoride and the effects on those who worked in the DuPont facility contracted as part of the Manhattan project, assembled by the University of Rochester, is presented in

Medical Experimentation During Cold War, The Plutonium Files: America's Secret Medical Experiments in the Cold War. Eileen Welsome, The Dial Press, 1999. Available at:
http://www.fluoridealert.org/p-files.htm
and *Fluoride, Teeth and the Atomic Bomb,*
http://www.fluoridealert.orgwastenot414.htm

Fluoride Toxicity: Your Teeth

Information about studies evaluating the effect of fluoride on the teeth, brain, and body of children and adults is available at the following sources:
http://www.fluoridealert.org/deepwater.htm

Peter Meiers. *The History of Fluorine, Fluoride and Fluoridation. Questionable Fluoride Safety Studies: Bartlett vs. Cameron & Newburgh vs. Kingston.* Available at:
http://www.fluoride-history.de/bartlett.htm

Fejerskov O, Richards A, DenBesten P. The effect of fluoride on tooth mineralization. In: Fejerskov O, Ekstrand J, Burt B, eds. *Fluoride in Dentistry, 2nd Edition.* Munksgaard, Copenhagen. 1996:112-152.

The following studies evaluated the effect of fluoride on organ systems:

Fejerskov O, Richards A, DenBesten P. The effect of fluoride on tooth mineralization. In: Fejerskov O, Ekstrand J, Burt B, eds. *Fluoride in Dentistry, 2nd Edition.* Munksgaard, Copenhagen. 1996:112-152.

Dr. Hardy Limeback, Head of Preventive Dentistry, University of Toronto. *Why I am now Officially Opposed to Adding Fluoride to Drinking Water.* 2000. Toronto, Ontario, Canada.

Environmental Working Group. *National Academy Calls for Lowering Fluoride Limits in Tap Water.* EWG news release, March 22, 2006. Available at: http://www.ewg.org/node/21000

Allen K, Agosta C, Estafan D. Using microabrasive material to remove fluorosis stains. *J Am Dent Assoc.* 2004;135:319-23.

Groth E. (1973). *Two Issues of Science and Public Policy: Air Pollution Control in the San Francisco Bay Area, and Fluoridation of Community Water Supplies* [PhD Dissertation]. Stanford University;1973.

National Research Council, Board on Environmental Studies and Toxicology (BEST). (2006). In: *Fluoride in Drinking Water: A Scientific Review of EPA's Standards.* Washington, DC: National Academies Press; 2006: page 13.

Information about the effect of fluoride on the structure of teeth is available in the following articles:

United States Department of Health & Human Services, Agency for Toxic Substances & Disease Registry [ATSDR]. *Toxicological profile for Fluorides, Hydrogen Fluoride, and Fluorine.* Atlanta, GA: US Department of Health and Human Services, Public Health Service;2003. Available at: http://www.atsdr.cdc.gov/toxprofiles/tp11.html

Aoba T, Fejerskov O. Dental fluorosis: chemistry and biology. *Crit Rev Oral Biol Med.* 2002;13:155-170.

DenBesten PK, Yan Y, Featherstone JD, Hilton JF, Smith CE, Li W. Effects of fluoride on rat dental enamel matrix proteinases. *Arch Oral Biol.* 2002;47:763-70.

Fomon, SJ, Ekstrand J, Ziegler EE. Fluoride intake and prevalence of dental fluorosis: trends in fluoride intake with special attention to infants. *J Public Health Dent.* 2000:60:131-139.

Sapov K, Gedalia I, Grobler S, Lewinstein I, Roman I, Shapira L, Hirschfeld Z, Teotia S. A laboratory assessment of enamel hypoplasia of teeth with varying severities of dental fluorosis. *J Oral Rehabil*, 1999;26: 672-627.

Burt BA, Eklund SA. In: *Dentistry, Dental Practice, and the Community*. 5th ed. Philadelphia, PA: WB Saunders Co; 1999.

Milan AM, Waddington RJ, Embery G. Altered phosphorylation of rat dentine phosphoproteins by fluoride in vivo. *Calcif Tissue Int*. 1999. 64: 234-238.

Fejerskov O, Manji F, Baelum V. The nature and mechanisms of dental fluorosis in man. *J Dent Res*. 1990;69:692-700.

Denbesten PK, Crenshaw MA, Wilson MH. Changes in the fluoride-induced modulation of maturation stage ameloblasts of rats. *J Dent Res*. 1985;64:1365-1370.

DenBesten PK, Crenshaw MA. The effects of chronic high fluoride levels on forming enamel in the rat. *Arch Oral Biol*. 1984;29:675-679.

Vieira A, Hancock R, Dumitriu M, Schwartz M, Limeback H, Grynpas M. How does fluoride affect dentin microhardness and mineralization? *J Dent Res*. 2005;84:951-957.

Fluoride and Sensitive Teeth: More a Cause than a Cure

The following article describes the effect of fluoride on the dentin of teeth:

Susheela AK, Bhatnagar M. Structural aberrations in fluorosed human teeth: Biochemical and scanning electron microscopic studies. *Arch Toxicol*. 1993; 67:573-79.

The following article describes the effect of fluoride on tooth sensitivity:

Vieira AP, Hancock R, Dumitriu M, Limeback H, Grynpas MD. Fluoride's effect on human dentin ultrasound velocity (elastic modulus) and tubule size. *Eur J Oral Sci*. 2006;114:83-88.

Fluoride: Simply Not Effective

Information about the Newburgh and Kingston study is available at the following web sites:

New York State Coalition Opposed to Fluoridation (NYSCOF). Fluoride No

Benefit to Low Income Children. Available at:
http://www.orgsites.com/ny/nyscof/_pgg2.php3

Peter Meiers. *The History of Fluorine, Fluoride and Fluoridation. Questionable Fluoride Safety Studies: Bartlett vs. Cameron & Newburgh vs. Kingston.* Available at:
http://www.fluoride-history.de/bartlett.htm

Information about the topical effect of fluoride is available from the following sources:

National Research Council, Board on Environmental Studies and Toxicology (BEST). (2006). In: *Fluoride in Drinking Water: A Scientific Review of EPA's Standards.* Washington, DC: National Academies Press;2006: page 13.

European Commission, Health & Consumer Protection Directorate-General, Scientific Committee on Consumer Products (SCCP). *The Safety of Fluorine Compounds in Oral Hygiene Products for Children Under the Age of six Years.* Adopted by the SCCP during the 5th plenary meeting, September 20, 2005. Available at:
http://ec.europa.eu/health/ph_risk/committees/04_sccp/docs/sccp_o_024.pdf

Hellwig E, Lennon AM. Systemic versus topical fluoride. *Caries Res.* 2004;38:258-262.

Warren JJ, Levy SM. Current and future role of fluoride in nutrition. *Dent Clin North Am.* 2003;47:225-243.

Brothwell D, Limeback H. Breastfeeding is protective against dental fluorosis in a nonfluoridated rural area of Ontario, Canada. *J Human Lactation.* 2003;19:386-390.

Aoba T, Fejerskov O. Dental fluorosis: chemistry and biology. *Crit Rev Oral Biol Med.* 2002;13(2):155-170.

Centers for Disease Control. *Recommendations for Using Fluoride to Prevent and Control Dental Caries in the United States.* MMWR. Aug 17, 2001;50(RR14):1-42. Available at:
http://www.cdc.gov/mmwr/preview/mmwrhtml/rr5014a1.htm

Featherstone, JDB. (2000). The Science and Practice of Caries Prevention. *J Am Dent Assoc.* 2000;131:887-899.

Formon SJ, Ekstrand J, Ziegler E. Fluoride Intake and Prevalence of Dental Fluorosis: Trends in Fluoride Intake with Special Attention to Infants. *J Pub Health Dent.* 2000;60:131-139.

Burt BA. The case for eliminating the use of dietary fluoride supplements for young children. *J Publ Health Dent*. 1999;59:260-274.

Featherstone JDB. (1999) Prevention and Reversal of Dental Caries: Role of Low Level Fluoride. *Com Dent & Oral Epidem*. 1999;27:31-40.

Adair SM. Overview of the history and current status of fluoride supplementation schedules. *J Public Health Dent*. 1999;59:252-258.

Limeback H. A re-examination of the pre-eruptive and post-eruptive mechanism of the anti-caries effects of fluoride: is there any anti-caries benefit from swallowing fluoride? *Community Dent Oral Epidemiol*.1999;27:62-71.

Diesendorf M, Colquhoun J, Spittle BJ, Everingham DN, Clutterbuck FW. New evidence on fluoridation. *Aust N Z J Public Health*. 1997;21:187-190.

Ekstrand J, Fomon SJ, Ziegler EE, Nelson SE. Fluoride pharmacokinetics in infancy. *Pediatr Res*.1994;35:157-163.

Zero DT, Raubertas RF, Fu J, Pedersen AM, Hayes AL, Featherstone JD. Fluoride concentrations in plaque, whole saliva, and ductal saliva after application of home-use topical fluorides [published erratum appears in J Dent Res 1993 Jan;72(1):87]. *J Dent Res*. 1992;71:1768-1775.

Wefel JS. Effects of fluoride on caries development and progression using intra-oral models. *J Dent Res*. 1990;69:626-633; discussion 634-626.

Fejerskov O, Thylstrup A, Larsen MJ. Rational use of fluorides in caries prevention. A concept based on possible cariostatic mechanisms. *Acta Odontol Scand*. 1981;39:241-249.

"[E]vidence has continued to accumulate to support the hypothesis that the anti-caries mechanism of fluoride is mainly a topical one."

Dr. Limeback's comment is available in *ADA Fluoridation Facts 2005*. Available at:

http://www.ada.org/public/topics/fluoride/facts/fluoridation_facts.pdf

The following case report describes the negative effect of fluoride solution on soft tissue and bone:

Sjostrom S, Kalfas S. Tissue necrosis after subgingival irrigation with fluoride solution. *J Clin Periodontol*. 1999;26:257-260.

The following study describes the rate of decay in two areas in the Sudan where fluoride levels in the drinking water varied 10-fold:

Ibrahim YE, Bjorvatn K, Birkeland JM. Caries and dental fluorosis in a 0.25 and a 2.5 ppm fluoride area in the Sudan. *Int J Paediatr Dent*. 1997;7:161-166.

The following document describes the rate of decay in Vancouver and Toronto, Canada:

ADA Fluoridation Facts 2005, available at: http://www.ada.org/public/topics/ fluoride/facts/fluoridation_facts.pdf

The following article reviewed 214 water fluoridation studies and was published in the British Medical Journal.

McDonagh MS, Whiting PF, Wilson PM, et al. Systematic review of water fluoridation. *Brit Med J.* 2000;321:855-859.

The abstract of the study addressing the effect of fluoride on the risk of dental decay by

Brian A. Burt, MPH, PhD of the University of Michigan was presented at the Dietary Fluoride Supplement Conference of the American Dental Association; the meeting was held in Chicago, Ill in January 1994.

The CDC Study

The location of tooth decay in children is described in the following documents:

Brown LJ, Kaste LM, Selwitz RH, Furman LJ. Dental caries and sealant usage in U.S. children, 1988-1991: selected findings from the Third National Health and Nutrition Examination Survey. *J Am Dent Assoc.* 1996;127:335-343.

Rethman J. Trends in preventive care: caries risk assessment and indications for sealants. *J Am Dent Assoc.* 2000;131 Suppl:8S-12S.

Pinkham JR, editor. *Pediatric dentistry: Infancy through adolescence.* 3rd ed. Philadelphia: Saunders; 1999.

White B. Toward Improving the Oral Health of Americans: an Overview of Oral Health Status, Resources and Care Delivery. *Public Health Reports.* 1993;108: 657-672.

Gray, AS. Fluoridation: Time for a New Base Line? *J Can Dent Assoc.* 1987;10:763-765.

The CDC report, *Surveillance for Dental Caries, Dental Sealants, Tooth Retention, Edentulism, and Enamel Fluorosis—United States, 1988-1994 and 1999-2002,* was published in MMWR. Aug 26, 2005.54(03);1-44. Available at: http://www.cdc.gov/mmwr/preview/mmwrhtml/ss5403a1.htm

The report, *Early Childhood Caries Trends Upward. Children's Dental Health Project,* 8 Sept 2005, is available at:
http://www.cdhp.org/downloads/mmwrfinal90805.pdf

Dental Fluorosis—How Severe and How Common?

Comment by Paul Connett, PhD, Professor of Chemistry at St. Lawrence University, Canton, NY, addressing the effect of fluoride on the human body is presented in the
New York State Coalition Opposed to Fluoridation (NYSCOF) document *Fluoride No Benefit to Low Income Children.* Available at:
http://www.orgsites.com/ny/nyscof/_pgg2.php3

The results of a British study evaluating the correlation between fluoridated water and dental fluorosis in children is reported by
Marian S McDonagh, Penny F Whiting, Paul M Wilson, Alex J Sutton, Ivor Chestnutt, Jan Cooper, Kate Misso, Matthew Bradley, Elizabeth Treasure, and Jos Kleijnen in "Systematic review of water fluoridation". *British Medical Journal.* 2000;321: 855-859; access at: doi:10.1136/bmj.321.7265.855

An update on a World Health Organization study, by
Wondwossen F, Astrøm AN, Bjorvatn K, Bårdsen A. The relationship between dental caries and dental fluorosis in areas with moderate- and high-fluoride drinking water in Ethiopia. *Community Dent Oral Epidemiol* 2004;32(5):337-44.

The results of a study, conducted at the Wales College of Medicine in the United Kingdom, which addressed the perceptions of individuals on images of other individuals who had dental fluorosis and dental caries is reported by
Williams DM, Chestnutt IG, Bennett PD, Hood K, Lowe R, Heard P. Attitudes to fluorosis and dental caries by a response latency method. *Community Dent Oral Epidemiol.* 2006;34:153-159.

The following studies, published since 1985, associate increasing tooth decay with fluorosis and two studies published in 2003 associate dental fluorosis with increases in dental caries, erosion, and tooth fracture.
Wondwossen F, Astrøm AN, Bjorvatn K, Bårdsen A. The relationship between dental caries and dental fluorosis in areas with moderate- and high-

fluoride drinking water in Ethiopia. *Community Dent Oral Epidemiol.* 2004;32(5):337-44.

Levy SM. An update on fluorides and fluorosis. *J Can Dent Assoc.* 2003;69:286-291.

Ekanayake L, van der Hoek W. Dental caries and developmental defects of enamel in relation to fluoride levels in drinking water in an arid area of Sri Lanka. *Caries Res.* 2002;36(6):398-404.

United States Department of Health & Human Services, Agency for Toxic Substances & Disease Registry [ATSDR]. *Toxicological profile for Fluorides, Hydrogen Fluoride, and Fluorine.* Atlanta, GA: US Department of Health and Human Services, Public Health Service;2003. Available at:
http://www.atsdr.cdc.gov/toxprofiles/tp11.html

Nanayakkara D, et al. Dental fluorosis and caries incidence in rural children residing in a high fluoride area in the dry zone of Sri Lanka. *Ceylon J Med Sci.* 1999;42:13-17.

Ibrahim YE, Bjorvatn K, Birkeland JM. Caries and dental fluorosis in a 0.25 and a 2.5 ppm fluoride area in the Sudan. *Int J Paediatr Dent.* 1997;7:161-166.

Cortes DF, Ellwood RP, O'Mullane DM, Bastos JR. Drinking water fluoride levels, dental fluorosis, and caries experience in Brazil. *J Public Health Dent.* 1996;56:226-228.

Mann J, Mahmoud W, Ernest M, Sgan-Cohen H, Shoshan N, Gedalia I. Fluorosis and dental caries in 6–8-year-old children in a 5 ppm fluoride area. *Community Dent Oral Epidemiol.* 1990;18:77-79.

Mann J, Tibi M, Sgan-Cohen HD. Fluorosis and caries prevalence in a community drinking above-optimal fluoridated water. *Community Dent Oral Epidemiol.* 1987;15:293-295.

Carlsson A. [Current problems of the pharmacology and toxicology of fluorides]. *Lakartidningen.* 1978;75:1388-1392.

Smith MC, Smith HV. (1940). Observations on the Durability of Mottled Teeth. *Am J Pub Health.* 1940;30:1050-1052.

ADA, Facts about Fluoride, available at:
http://www.ada.org/public/topics/fluoride/fluoride_article01.asp

Fluoride Toxicity: the Whole Body

More information from the report by the Public Health Engineering Department in India which investigated villages in regions known to have high levels of fluoride in the water is available through

Infochange Health in India, Jan 2003 and is available at
http://www.infochangeindia.org/
    searcharchives.jsp?recordno=1941&secno=2&detail=T
Now available at:
http://infochangeindia.org/component/option,com_joomap/Itemid,131

The results of a study demonstrating the effect of fluoride on a specific cellular pathway in an animal model is reported by Li and associates in

Li Y, Decker S, Yuan ZA, et al. Effects of sodium fluoride on the actin cytoskeleton of murine ameloblasts. *Arch Oral Biol*. 2005;50:681–688.

The results of a study demonstrating the effect of fluoride on dentin mineralization in an in vitro model is reported by Moseley and associates.

Moseley R, Waddington RJ, Sloan AJ, Smith AJ, Hall RC, Embery G. The influence of fluoride exposure on dentin mineralization using an in vitro organ culture model. *Calcif Tissue Int*. 2003;73:470–475.

The results of studies demonstrating that fluoride can induce programmed cell death to occur early and can cause changes in cell reproduction in animal models is reported by

Le and Chen. DNA damage, apoptosis and cell cycle changes induced by fluoride in rat oral mucosal cells and hepatocytes. *World J Gastroenterol*. 2006;12:1144–1148.

The results of studies examining the influence of fluoride human embryo liver cells are reported by Wang and associates.

Wang AG, Xia T, Chu QL, et al. Effects of fluoride on lipid peroxidation, DNA damage and apoptosis in human embryo hepatocytes. *Biomed Environ Sci*. 2004;17:217–222.

The results of studies examining the effects of fluoride and selenium on liver cells is reported by Wang and associates.

Effects of selenium and fluoride on apoptosis and lipid peroxidation in human hepatocytes, (Article in Chinese) *Zhonghua Yu Fang Yi Xue Za Zhi*. 2002;36:235–238.

More of Dr. Limeback's comments on the effect of fluoride on the body are available in

ADA Fluoridation Facts 2005, available at:

http://www.ada.org/public/topics/fluoride/facts/fluoridation_facts.pdf

The following studies examined the influence of fluoride on bone.

Hillier S, Cooper C, Kellingray S, Russell G, Hughes H, Coggon D. Fluoride in drinking water and risk of hip fracture in the UK: a case-control study. *Lancet.* 2000;355:265-269.

Alhava EM, Olkkonen H, Kauranen P, Kari T. The effect of drinking water fluoridation on the fluoride content, strength and mineral density of human bone. *Acta Orthop Scand.* 1980;51:413-420.

Arnala I. *Bone fluoride, histomorphometry and incidence of hip fracture.* University of Kuopio, Kuopio 1983.

Arnala I, Alhava EM, Kauranen P. Effects of fluoride on bone in Finland. Histomorphometry of cadaver bone from low and high fluoride areas. *Acta Orthop Scand.* 1980;56:161-166.

The results of a study examining the effect of drinking water which contains naturally occurring high levels of fluoride on the body is reported by

Alarcon-Herrera and associates. Well water fluoride, dental fluorosis, bone fractures in the Guadiana Valley of Mexico. *Fluoride.* 2001;34:139-149.

The results of a study, conducted in the USA, which examined the relationship between fluoridated drinking water and risk of wrist fracture is reported by

Phipps KR, Orwoll ES, Mason JD, Cauley JA. Community water fluoridation, bone mineral density, and fractures: prospective study of effects in older women. *Brit Med J.* 2000;321:860-864.

Additional information collected in the initial Newburgh-Kingston Study which addresses safety issues related to fluoride use is available at:

http://fluoridedangers.blogspot.com/2006/01/human-experiment-predicts-fluoride.html

National Research Council, Subcommittee on Health Effects of Ingested Fluoride. In: *Health effects of ingested fluoride.* Washington, DC: National Academy Press;1993: pages 73-74.

The following studies examine the relationship between fluoride and bone strength:

Alhava EM, Olkkonen H, Kauranen P, Kari T. The effect of drinking water fluoridation on the fluoride content, strength and mineral density of human bone. *Acta Orthop Scand*. 1980;51:413-420.

Bayley TA, Harrison JE, Murray TM, et al. Fluoride-induced fractures: relation to osteogenic effect. *J Bone Miner Res*. 1990;5 Suppl 1:S217-222.

Carter DR, Beaupre GS. Effects of fluoride treatment on bone strength. *J Bone Miner Res*. 1990;5 Suppl 1:S177-184.

A study conducted by Danielson and colleagues reported a higher incidence of hip fracture in individuals exposed to fluoridated drinking water.

Danielson C, Lyon JL, Egger M, Goodenough GK. Hip fractures and fluoridation in Utah's elderly population. *JAMA*. 1992;268:746-748.

The following studies address fluoride-induced changes in bone:

Riggs BL, O'Fallon WM, Lane A, et al. Clinical trial of fluoride therapy in postmenopausal osteoporotic women: extended observations and additional analysis. *J Bone Miner Res*. 1994;9:265-275.

Sowers MF, Clark MK, Jannausch ML, Wallace RB. A prospective study of bone mineral content and fracture in communities with differential fluoride exposure. *Am J Epidemiol*. 1991;133:649-660.

Sowers MR, Wallace RB, Lemke JH. The relationship of bone mass and fracture history to fluoride and calcium intake: a study of three communities. *Am J Clin Nutr*. 1986;44:889-898.

The following studies, conducted in Finland, address the relationship between fluoridated water and damage to bone structure:

Carter DR, Beaupre GS. Effects of fluoride treatment on bone strength. *J Bone Miner Res*. 1990;5 Suppl 1:S177-184.

Arnala I, Alhava EM, Kauranen P. Effects of fluoride on bone in Finland. Histomorphometry of cadaver bone from low and high fluoride areas. *Acta Orthop Scand*. 1985;56:161-166.

Arnala I, Alhava EM, Kivivuori R, Kauranen P. Hip fracture incidence not affected by fluoridation: Osteofluorosis studied in Finland. *Acta Orthop Scand*. 1986;57:344-348.

The results of a study attempting to examine the long-term effects of fluoride on bone health is reported by Alhava and associates.

Alhava EM, Olkkonen H, Kauranen P, Kari T. The effect of drinking water fluoridation on the fluoride content, strength and mineral density of human bone. *Acta Orthopaedica Scandinavica.* 1980;51(3):413-420.

The following studies address the influence of fluoride on bone at different stages of life:

Danielson C, Lyon JL, Egger M, Goodenough GK. Hip fractures and fluoridation in Utah's elderly population. *JAMA.* 1992;268:746-748.

Riggs BL, Hodgson SF, O'Fallon WM, et al. Effect of fluoride treatment on the fracture rate in postmenopausal women with osteoporosis. *N Engl J Med.* 1990;322:802-809.

The following studies address the relationship between bone mass and bone strength:

Bayley TA, Harrison JE, Murray TM, et al. Fluoride-induced fractures: relation to osteogenic effect. *J Bone Miner Res.* 1990;5 Suppl 1:S217-222.

Carter DR, Beaupre GS. Effects of fluoride treatment on bone strength. *J Bone Miner Res.* 1990;5 Suppl 1:S177-184.

Riggs BL, Hodgson SF, O'Fallon WM, et al. Effect of fluoride treatment on the fracture rate in postmenopausal women with osteoporosis. *N Engl J Med.* 1990;322(12):802-809.

The following studies address the influence of hormones and hormone production on bone health:

Brodowska A. [The influence of hormonal replacement therapy on bone density in postmenopausal women depending on polymorphism of vitamin D receptor (VDR) and estrogen receptor (ER) genes]. *Ann Acad Med Stetin.* 2003;49:111-130.

Berenson AB, Breitkopf CR, Grady JJ, Rickert VI, Thomas A. Effects of hormonal contraception on bone mineral density after 24 months of use. *Obstet Gynecol.* 2004;103(5 Pt 1):899-906.

Borer KT. Physical activity in the prevention and amelioration of osteoporosis in women : interaction of mechanical, hormonal and dietary factors. *Sports Med.* 2005;35:779-830.

Paschalis EP, Burr DB, Mendelsohn R, Hock JM, Boskey AL. Bone mineral and collagen quality in humeri of ovariectomized cynomolgus monkeys given rhPTH(1-34) for 18 months. *J Bone Miner Res.* 2003;18:769-775.

Abrams SA. Normal acquisition and loss of bone mass. *Horm Res.* 2003;60 Suppl 3:71–76.

Dr. Bassin's research addressing the association between exposure to fluoride and risk of cancer is presented in

Bassin EB, Wypij D, Davis RB, Mittleman MA. Age-specific fluoride exposure in drinking water and osteosarcoma (United States). *Cancer Causes Control.* 2006;17:421–428.

More information on the closed-door hearing of Dr. Chester Douglass by the Harvard Ethics Panel and Dr. Chester Douglass' subsequent gifts to Harvard University Dental School is available at:

www.ewg.org search Chester Douglass

http://www.ewg.org/node/18801

http://www.ewg.org/node/18566

http://www.ewg.org/node/8761

http://www.ewg.org/node/20997

Index

A

A.E.I. duPont du Nemours Company 144
Accutherm 71
Agency for Toxic Substances and Disease Registry
69, 108, 126, 277, 278, 280, 284–
287, 295, 298, 299. *See* mercury
Alice in Wonderland 24
alpha lipoic acid 90
Alzheimer's disease 24, 104, 126, 266, 297
amalgam alloy. *See* mercury
American Academy of Pediatrics
37, 191, 203, 206, 278
American Conference of Governmental Industrial Hyg
69, 128, 285
American Dental Association
23, 43, 46, 47, 51, 52, 80, 98, 99, 117,
134, 140, 141, 149, 151, 154, 184–
187, 190, 192, 193, 206, 209, 233,
280, 303, 309
American Society of Dental Surgeons
22, 23, 48, 275
ANSI 129
antioxidant 89, 90, 93, 181, 293
Ast, David 146, 303
atomic absorption spectrometer 60
Atomic Energy Commission 146
atopic eczema 103
ATSDR. *See* Agency for Toxic Substances and Disease
Registry
attenuated cultures 38
autoimmune thyroiditis 103

B

Baltimore College of Dental Surgery 22
Barnett, Henry 148
Best Management Practices 43
BioSafeDentistry™ 7
blood urea/nitrogen (BUN) 105
blood-brain barrier 104
Bryson, Chris 143

C

California Superior Court 28
carcinogen 30, 71, 126, 127, 129

Cardiovascular System 100, 295
Carroll, Lewis 24
Center for Disease Control 46, 126, 189, 285
chelation. *See* Protocols
children 9, 12, 26, 32, 38, 51, 55, 70–
72, 83, 92, 102, 108, 133, 134, 138,
140, 142, 144, 147, 149, 154–
158, 161–164, 169, 170, 176, 178,
180, 186–197, 201–205, 206–
211, 212, 220, 221, 244, 272,
284, 291, 298, 304, 306–310
chlorella (www.vitacost.com) 91
Christian Science Monitor 143
chronic fatigue 21, 101, 103, 267
coal-fired power plants 33, 278, 294
Code of Federal Regulations 37, 54, 207
color confusion index (CCI) 106
Colorado brown stain 144
Consumers for Dental Choice 99
coproporphyrinogen oxidase [CPOX4]) 99
Council on Dental Materials, Instruments and Equip
42, 117
creatinine 105
Cremation Association of North America 33
cremations 33
Crohn's disease. *See* gastrointestinal
crowns
gold 112, 114, 115, 121, 242
metal 112, 122, 124, 128
metals 244
porcelain 117

D

decayed, missing and filled teeth (DMF) 147
Deepwater 144, 146, 303, 304
Denclude toothpaste 212, 213
dental amalgam fillings. *See* mercury
dental tattoo 76, 77, 287
Department of Health and Human Services
11, 31, 32, 95, 108, 177, 283, 286, 305, 311
Detroit Water and Sewerage Department 42
DMPS (2,3-dimercaptopropane-1-sulfonate)
73, 74, 81, 82, 282, 289
DMSA (meso-2,3-dimercaptosuccinic acid) 60, 74
DuPont 31, 145, 146, 149, 156, 276, 304

317

About the Author

Donald Robbins received his doctorate of medical dentistry from the University of Pennsylvania School of Dental Medicine at a young age and has continued to train throughout his career. He is a current fellow of the Academy of General Dentistry and an associate of the International Academy for Oral Medicine and Toxicology and a former fellow of the International College of Cranio-Mandibular Orthopedics and diplomat of the American Academy of Pain Management.

Following graduation in 1973, Dr. Robbins taught at the University of Pennsylvania School of Dental Medicine and began practicing dentistry in the private office setting. Since 1982, he has practiced biologic dentistry, eliminating the use of mercury and other hazardous materials from the treatments he has provided to patients. During the last 10 years, he has developed the BioSafeDentistry system, which employs no mercury, fluoride, or other toxic chemicals and materials and so allows dentists to protect the overall health of their patients. He has endeavored to teach this dental practice system to other dentists wishing to improve patient care in their own offices. In recent years he has conducted a practice-based research program that has demonstrated the connection between silver/mercury dental fillings and on-going mercury levels in individuals exposed to those fillings.

Dr. Robbins has developed a technical training program for those entering a career in dental assisting. He established a private school licensed by the State of Pennsylvania and taught the program at his school, The Dental Training Center, for four years. In 2007, he joined forces with Delaware County Community College in southeastern Pennsylvania to offer his training program to more students. He serves as director of the program, which graduates more than 25 students each year as dental assistants.

Marquis Book Printing Inc.

Québec, Canada
2009